THE BACH
REMEDIES
WORKBOOK

By the same author

Bach Flower Remedies for Men

THE BACH REMEDIES WORKBOOK

STEFAN BALL

Illustrated by Paul Margiotta

Index compiled by Mary Kirkness

SAFFRON WALDEN
THE C.W. DANIEL COMPANY LIMITED

This edition first published in Great Britain in 1998
by The C. W. Daniel Company Limited
1 Church Path, Saffron Walden,
Essex, CB10 1JP, United Kingdom

© Stefan Ball 1998

ISBN 0 85207 311 9

Designed by Jim Reader.
Designed and produced in association with
Book Production Consultants plc, Cambridge, England.
Typeset by Cambridge Photosetting Services, Cambridge, England.
Printed in England by Hillman Printers (Frome), Ltd. England.

FOR
GRACE VERA FARRANT

CONTENTS

Introduction   11

Acknowledgements   17

Day 1   Mood Remedies   19

Day 2   Everyday Emergencies   43

Day 3   Type Remedies   63

Day 4   The Holistic Approach   85

Day 5   Healing Yourself   103

Day 6   Healing Others   121

Day 7   Putting it all Together   147

         Where to Go from Here   173

         Appendix   181

         Index   187

INTRODUCTION

Before we start ...

Five of the seven dwarves have managed to catch a cold in the diamond mines. They ask the sixth dwarf, Dopey, to suggest a cure for them. He says there's no cure for a cold and they'll just have to stick it out until it's gone.

So they ask the seventh dwarf, Doc, who has just finished working through this book. He gives four of them a single flower remedy from Dr Bach's system, but each remedy is different. As you work through the book yourself, see if you can work out which remedy each dwarf got, and what happened to the fifth dwarf.

> **FIVE DWARVES**
>
> In case you've forgotten, Walt Disney named our five cold-ridden dwarves: Happy, Sleepy, Sneezy, Bashful and Grumpy.

This book and its readers

This book is about a complete system of 38 remedies which balance emotions and treat negative mental states. It is also about the man who discovered them, Dr Edward Bach, and his unique approach to healing. It is a self-study course in the remedies and their use, and as such helps to realise one of Dr Bach's dearest wishes, that people should learn how to take control of their own health.

There are already a number of excellent reference books on Dr Bach and his work, not least Dr Bach's own *The Twelve Healers*. Seminars and workshops take place all over the world and special courses for professional practitioners are run under the auspices of the Dr Edward Bach Foundation. This book could not and does not replace these other approaches, but augments them. It is written for beginners and near-beginners, and seeks to provide the building blocks that people need if they are to start discovering the remedies for themselves. It assumes no knowledge, but in seven short chapters covers all 38 of the Bach Flower Remedies and the states of mind and emotions that they can be used to

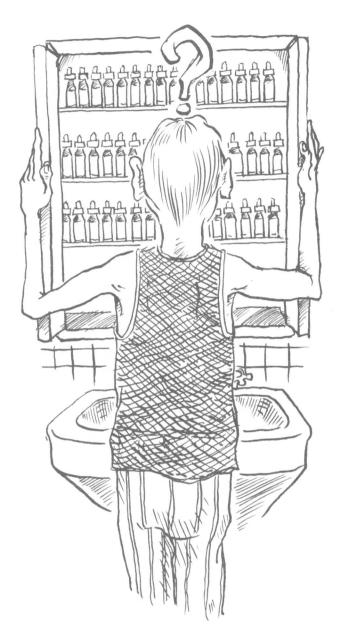

help. The aim has been to provide enough information and practical exercises to enable anyone to gain a comprehensive grasp of Dr Bach's work. After following this course readers should be able to help themselves, their friends and their relations, and will be well prepared for any further training in the use of the remedies that they intend to undertake.

How the book is structured.

Dr Bach wanted a system that would be easy to use, and I hope that by the time you have completed this course you will agree that he succeeded. Nevertheless there is one great difficulty that new-comers to the remedies face right at the outset. This is the fact that there are 38 remedies to learn, and for each remedy a different set of indications. This can appear a formidable hurdle.

This system of treatment is the most perfect which has been given to mankind within living memory.

THE TWELVE HEALERS AND OTHER REMEDIES

I have tried to smooth your way as much as possible by approaching the problem in three complementary ways. First of all, in each of the seven chapters a different group of remedies is discussed in detail, and exercises are devised specifically to reinforce those remedies. At the same time you will find that other exercises refer back to remedies that were mentioned in previous chapters, so helping to keep old knowledge fresh in your mind. Finally, and right from the first chapter, there are questions which call for a knowledge of remedies that you have not yet covered. When you reach an exercise like this you will find either a brief explanation of what these 'new' remedies are for, or explicit instructions to refer to the list of remedies in the Appendix. In most cases I have tried also to restrict the number of remedies you have to choose from.

All know that the same disease may have different effects on different people: it is the effects that need treatment, because they guide to the real cause.

THE TWELVE HEALERS AND OTHER REMEDIES

Don't worry too much about this – all will become clear as you work through the book.

To find the answers to an exercise look on the next page – there's no need to turn the book upside down or keep your finger stuck in the back. Where the questions involve remedy selection I have tried to anticipate the wrong answers that might be given and explain them in the answer. Don't be afraid to make mistakes, then, because they are just as much a part of learning as selecting correctly. And if you really don't understand why something is wrong – or right – and I haven't covered it, phone the Dr Edward Bach Centre and ask. (See the Appendix for the number.)

The main reason for the failure of modern medical science is that is dealing with results and not causes.

HEAL THYSELF

As well as the remedy descriptions and exercises, each chapter contains background information on Dr Bach and his work. There are also projects which encourage you to use the remedies and to think more deeply about them and about yourself – look for the 'Hands-On' heading. Finally, a 'Quick Quiz' rounds off each chapter, just so that you can convince yourself that you really have been learning.

What you need before you start

As I've said, you do not need to know anything about Dr Bach's work to start using this book. And you certainly don't need to go out and buy all 38 of the remedies before you begin. You will find it useful to have a bottle of Rescue Remedy, though, and one or two stock bottles – in other words, single remedies bought from a chemist or health food shop. You might get a bottle of Olive and one of White Chestnut, or just look through the list of the remedies in the Appendix and buy the one or two that seem to strike a particular chord with you.

Apart from that you just need an open mind and a desire to learn. And a basic curiosity about who you are and how you feel. Because this book is really all about you.

About the author

I've written two books on this subject before, and I've been a full-time consultant at the Dr Edward Bach Centre since March 1996. I'm involved in developing and presenting the Practitioner Course and in all other aspects of the Centre's work, including the vital work of making the mother tinctures.

On a more mundane level my background also includes a couple of years spent developing course materials for a computer training company and a degree in languages. As a courseware developer and a language student I saw lots of workbooks and self-study courses, from the inspiring to the awful. I've tried to learn from failures and successes alike to make this course interesting and fun to use. If you don't think I succeeded I'd be happy to hear about it so I can do a better job next time around.

ACKNOWLEDGEMENTS

You don't need to read this bit unless you really want to, but I would be very remiss if I didn't acknowledge the very great help I have received – much of it unwitting – in preparing this book.

Above all I need to thank my wife Christine and daughters Alexandra and Madeleine, who keep me sane and remind me there is a world beyond the computer screen. Great thanks also to John Ramsell and Judy Howard for inviting me to join the Mount Vernon team, to Kathy Nicholson for pointing out what I should be looking for, and of course to Muriel Ramsell, Jackie Charles and Keith Howard. Our debt to Edward Bach himself, and to Nora Weeks and Victor Bullen, who were his successors and our predecessors, is beyond simple acknowledgement.

Karen Chapman, Dominique Le Bourgeois, Lynn Macwhinnie, Paula Crabtree and Eleanore Loos talked about teaching the Bach Flower Remedies while I gained the benefit of their experience. Other teachers, trainers and would-be trainers who I met over the years also helped enormously, long before this book was planned.

A special thank you for services above and beyond the call of duty goes to Judy Howard and Karen Chapman, who read through this work in draft and gave me their honest comments and suggestions. The fault for any mistakes that have dodged their careful editing is of course my own.

At the risk of becoming long-winded I'd also like to record debts of various magnitude to the Microsoft Corporation, Helen Morgan, Mr Valentine and the BBC. If I've forgotten anyone I can only apologise. It's in the nature of things that the biggest debts always go unpaid.

Day 1

MOOD REMEDIES

Hands on

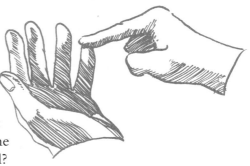

How do you feel at the moment? Is there anything worrying you? Are you under stress, or are you relaxed? Are you happy? Do you feel in control, or are things running away from you? What are your feelings? When was the last time you stopped to think about how you feel?

Close the book for a minute and think about it.

What the remedies do

There are 38 Bach Flower Remedies, and each one of them is aimed at a different state of mind or emotion. They do not treat physical illness directly, but by restoring harmony to the mind they allow the body's natural defences to work more easily. This means that people can quite literally heal themselves.

Dr Bach worked in the first three decades of our century. Today there are things in our lives that he knew nothing about, such as AIDS, large-scale environmental damage and repetitive strain injury. But the emotions these things provoke are no different from the emotions provoked in Dr Bach's day: we are scared of AIDS, full of righteous indignation at the harm done to our planet and worried about RSI.

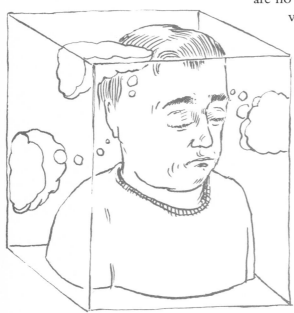

Dr Bach's system is complete because it treats emotions and not the triggers that cause them. It is not just for today, yesterday or tomorrow, but for all time.

Exercise 1a

See if you can match the seven remedies listed below with the moods described. Turn the page for the answers.

REMEDIES

1. Holly (the remedy for negative feelings towards others, such as hatred, jealousy, suspicion and spite)

2. Mimulus (the remedy for everyday fear and anxiety caused by known things; also for shyness and timidity)

3. Vervain (the remedy for over-enthusiasm in the name of a cause)

4. Hornbeam (the remedy for tiredness at the thought of the tasks that lie ahead)

5. Impatiens (the remedy for impatience)

6. Walnut (the remedy for protection against change and outside influences)

7. White Chestnut (the remedy for constant, repetitive, worrying thoughts)

MOODS

a. You can feel your stomach in a knot as you stand in the queue at the bank. You've got a meeting in 10 minutes and the clerks seem to be working slowly on purpose.

b. You wake up in the morning more tired than when you went to bed.

Fortunately once you manage to drag yourself out of bed and get started you find your energy returns bit by bit.

c. You can't forgive your ex-wife for betraying you with that man: you're jealous, yes, but more than that you hate the sight of the pair of them – and you don't mind if they know it.

d. As part of your new job you have to go for a routine x-ray. You're worrying all the time about what the x-ray might or might not show, and you find it hard to think about anything else.

e. You've been told you need to take a holiday – but there's so much still to do, and with the election coming up and all those campaign letters to write you won't have any time to spare for a long time to come.

f. You had an argument with a neighbour a few days ago and now you're frightened of running into him again.

g. You've just moved to a new neighbourhood. You feel unsettled and out of place where you are now.

Answers to Exercise 1a

MOOD a	needs	REMEDY 5.
MOOD b	needs	REMEDY 4.
MOOD c	needs	REMEDY 1.
MOOD d	needs	REMEDY 7.
MOOD e	needs	REMEDY 3.
MOOD f	needs	REMEDY 2.
MOOD g	needs	REMEDY 6.

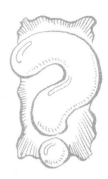

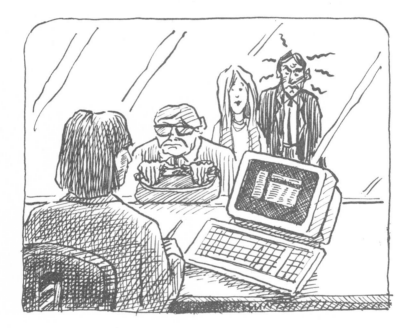

Remedies for Fear

Dr Bach grouped his 38 remedies under seven headings. Each of the seven chapters in this book features one of the groups. The first one we will deal with contains the remedies for different types of fear.

MIMULUS

- 'Our neighbours have a large dog that barks at me when I go past their gate. It always makes me jump and it's got so I dread going home in case it's there.'

We are all ready to admit the many results which may follow a fit of violent temper, the shock of sudden bad news; if trivial affairs can thus affect the body, how much more serious and deep-rooted must be a prolonged conflict between soul and body.

HEAL THYSELF

- 'I've got to give a speech next week and I feel really anxious about it.'

- 'I've got a lump in my breast but I'm scared of going to the doctor because of what he might say.'

- 'Hospitals always give me the willies.'

Mimulus is the remedy for normal, everyday fears and anxieties. Mimulus fears are *known* fears because sufferers know why they are afraid — they can name a cause.

Mimulus is also associated with people who tend to be shy and timid in all they do.

The positive quality of the Mimulus remedy is to provide a simple courage that allows the person to face the everyday problems of life without being deflected by anxiety.

RED CHESTNUT

- 'It may look silly, but I'd sooner drive down and pick my son up than have him coming home by himself on the train. He may be eighteen, but you only have to look at the papers to see what can happen.'

— CASE HISTORY —

It's a sunny day, and Brian has just kissed his wife and children goodbye and is off to a job that he really likes very much indeed. Suddenly, and for no reason, an uneasy conviction comes over him: something awful is about to happen.

- Aspen for his motiveless fear and sense of foreboding.

- 'Jane has gone abroad. She's with her friends, I suppose, but I won't be able to relax until she gets home.'

- 'Alice has had a couple of headaches recently. She says it's because she's been working too long on the computer, but I keep telling her to see the doctor, just in case.'

Mimulus fears are typically centred on what might happen to *you* – but where the fear is about what might happen to a loved one there is a different remedy to take. This is Red Chestnut, which works to calm exaggerated fears for our children, husbands, wives and parents, so that we can send out signals of calm and support to people in insecure situations, rather than terrifying them with our own fears.

ASPEN

- 'There's something about this place that makes me jumpy.'

- 'I just feel as if something awful is going to happen.'

- 'I can be in the middle of a conversation when suddenly I start shaking. There's no reason for it and I try telling myself not to be silly. But it's no good – I'm looking all around to find what's frightening me when there's nothing to be scared of.'

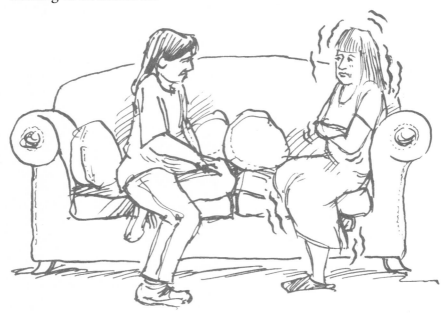

With both Mimulus and Red Chestnut sufferers can easily name a cause for the way they feel. The Aspen fear is different, however, for it is a vague fear, with no known, rational cause.

The positive action of Aspen is to calm this uncanny fear so that the person can face the real world with more confidence.

ROCK ROSE

- 'The car almost hit me. I was shaking so much I had to sit down there in the road.'

- 'Thomas woke the house with his screams. I don't know what he was dreaming about but he was frightened half to death.'

Rock Rose is the remedy for terror. It can be seen as an extension of the Mimulus and Aspen states – in other words, both known and unknown fears can be treated with Rock Rose where there is real terror rather than simple fear or anxiety.

CHERRY PLUM

- 'If this goes on I'm going to crack. I'll end up doing myself in or something.'

- 'It's driving me mad.'

Cherry Plum is the remedy for a very particular kind of fear: the fear of losing one's self-control and of doing harm to oneself or to someone else. People in the Cherry Plum state may be in some desperation, because they can feel their control going. They are frightened of what they might do; they may talk of suicide or appear hysterical or violent. The Cherry Plum remedy can be thought of as a tonic for the reason, allowing the individual to master his mind and act quietly to solve his problems rather than giving way beneath the burden.

– CASE HISTORY –

After seeing a scary film on TV, eight-year-old Darren wakes in the night screaming.

- Rock Rose for the terror of the dream – or Rescue Remedy.

MEDICAL BACKUP

The Bach Flower Remedies can be used in conjunction with other forms of treatment or therapy. This fact should be borne in mind whenever there are definite physical or psychological symptoms. In particular anyone talking of suicide should be taken seriously, and professional help should be sought at once from a doctor or other qualified professional.

Exercise 1b

Fill in the blanks in these statements.

1. If you are scared of losing control and doing yourself some harm, you need

    _____.

2.. If you are frightened of something you can name, you need

    _____.

3. If you feel anxious but you can't put your finger on the cause of you anxiety, you need

    _____.

4. If you are fearful of something happening to someone that you care about, you need

    _____.

5. If you are truly terrified you need

    _____.

Answers to Exercise 1b

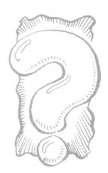

1. Cherry Plum

2. Mimulus

3. Aspen

4. Red Chestnut

5. Rock Rose

Who was Dr Bach?

Dr Edward Bach, MB, BS, MRCS, LRCP, DPH, was a consultant pathologist, bacteriologist and homoeopath. He was born in 1886 in Moseley, just outside Birmingham, although the origins of the family probably lay in Wales. He began studying medicine in 1906 at Birmingham University, moving later to University College, London, where he completed his studies in 1912.

He was turned down for service in the First World War because of his ill-health, but despite this he undertook many extra duties during the war so as to help care for the injured. These responsibilities, in addition to his researches, caused him to overwork and led to a collapse in 1917. The surgeons who operated on him said that he had only three months to live, so as soon as he could he threw himself back into his work in the hope that he would be able to make some lasting contribution to medicine before his death. But as the months went by he found himself growing stronger and concluded that this was because he was happy and inspired by his work.

For Bach, the belief that mental states could have a direct and powerful effect on physical health was confirmed by this experience. When he discovered

SAINT BACH?

People have on occasion tried to put Dr Bach on a pedestal, but in fact he was in many respects a very ordinary person. He liked country walks and a sing-song in the local pub. He dug his own garden at Mount Vernon and made his own rough-and-ready furniture. Those who knew him have told how at times he could be irritable, short-tempered and not at all saintly, just like everyone else. In fact it was because he shared the normal faults of ordinary people that he was able to sympathise with and understand them so well.

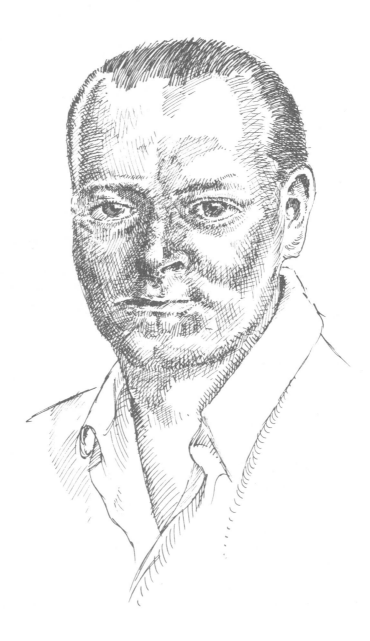

A fuller account of Dr Bach's life and researches can be found in Nora Weeks's book *The Medical Discoveries of Edward Bach, Physician*. See the chapter 'Where to Go from Here' for more details.

Hahnemann's writings on homoeopathy he felt that he was at last on the road to the natural treatment he wanted to find.

Eventually he abandoned his successful and lucrative Harley Street practice. He devoted himself full-time to his new system of medicine that would help people as individuals instead of simply treating their symptoms. Over the next five years he completed the series of 38 remedies and a year after that, in 1936, he died. It was as if his constant researches provided the spark that kept him going, and once the work was complete his life too had reached a natural end-point.

Taking a Remedy

There are a couple of ways to take the Bach Flower Remedies. The simplest, which is most often used for passing moods, is to take them in a glass of water. Try this now:

STOCK BOTTLES

'Stock bottle' is the name given to the bottle of concentrated remedy that you buy in a shop.

1. Put some water into a glass or cup (it doesn't matter how much water you put in)

2. Select a stock bottle containing a single remedy that you want to take and use the dropper in the bottle top to add 2 drops of it to the water

3. Add further remedies as required, up to six or seven different ones

OTHER WAYS TO TAKE THE REMEDIES

You can also make up treatment bottles for more convenient long-term use or take the remedies externally in an emergency. See later on in this chapter for how to make up a treatment bottle; external use is covered in Day 2.

That's all there is to it. If you were actually using this remedy mix, you would simply sip from the glass until the feelings you are treating have passed. If you were treating a more long-standing problem then you should sip from the glass at least four times a day — but more often if you feel you need to — and make up a fresh glass each day.

You might think that something so simple would hardly need practising, but it's surprising how often people get confused over dosage.

In most of us there is one, or more, adverse defect which is particularly hindering our advancement, and it is such a defect, or defects, which we must especially seek out within ourselves ...

HEAL THYSELF

Exercise 1c

Which fear remedy or remedies do the following people need? Try to do the exercise from memory alone, then check your answers in the following section.

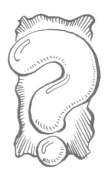

1.   'It's when the baby won't stop crying that it gets to me. I just lose it. I'm terrified that one day I'll really snap and who knows what I'll do.'

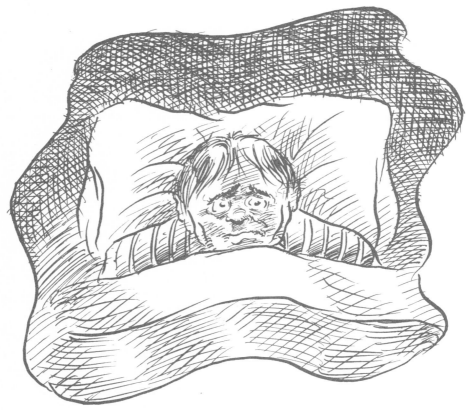

... not only must physical means be used, choosing always the best methods which are known to the art of healing, but we ourselves must also endeavour to the utmost of our ability to remove any fault in our nature; because final and complete healing ultimately comes from within ...

HEAL THYSELF

2. 'It's not confidence. I know I can drive. But every time I get behind the wheel I start worrying about hitting someone or crashing into a lamppost or something.'

3. 'I keep getting these nightmares where I'm being chased, and I wake up with my hair literally standing on end and the bedclothes all in a heap. After that it takes ages to get back to sleep. I just lie there in the dark with the horrors.'

4. 'He's already had one attack but he won't slow down. I keep expecting the worst. You could say that his health problems are making me ill.'

5. 'I just know there's something terribly wrong in my life, and it frightens me to death. But I can't put my finger on what it is. I suppose an outsider would say there's nothing wrong.'

6. 'When I heard there had been a crash I just went into a blind panic.'

What we know as disease is the terminal stage of a much deeper disorder.

HEAL THYSELF

COMBINATION REMEDIES

Responsible pharmacists do not sell 'ready-mixed' bottles of remedies for specific problems, because different individuals faced with the same situations will need different remedies according to their different personalities and the way they react to the same conditions.

There is, however, one combination remedy which Dr Bach himself formulated, and which is used against the emotions commonly aroused by crises and emergencies. This is known as Rescue Remedy, and as you might expect, it contains both Rock Rose, for terror, and Cherry Plum for loss of self control.

There is more about Rescue Remedy in the next chapter.

Answers to exercise 1c

1. Cherry Plum is the remedy specifically for the fear that you might lose control of yourself and do something awful.

2. This person uses the word 'worry', so you might have considered White Chestnut if you were looking in the list at the back of the book (and if you forgot that you were only looking for fear remedies). But the person is not worrying all the time, which *would* indicate White Chestnut, rather she is suffering from a specific, named anxiety that comes under specific, named conditions – in other words, when she gets behind the wheel of a car. This is a Mimulus fear.

3. Rock Rose is for terror, and this would certainly be the correct remedy to give when this person first wakes up after the nightmare. But you might also consider Aspen for the vague, uncanny fears that keep him from getting to sleep again afterwards. With luck, though, prompt treatment with Rock Rose would calm him enough so that the Aspen state would not arise in the first place.

4. This is a Red Chestnut fear. Even if the first person's fears for the second person's health are justified they are not helping the situation. They are only making the worrier as ill as the person being worried over.

5. This is Aspen: a fear with no known cause.

6. Rock Rose is the remedy for terror, but as there seems also to have been a loss of self-control you might consider Cherry Plum as well. This is for the fear of losing one's self-control, of course, but it can also be given when control has in fact been lost – in other words when the feared event has actually happened.

The true cause of disease

Orthodox medicine is fairly clear about what causes most diseases. It is something external to the individual. So influenza and cold sores are caused by viruses, thrush is caused by a fungus and asthma has a number of possible causes including pollution and allergies.

The question Dr Bach asked himself was why only some of the people exposed to these agents of disease went on to fall ill. He suggested that in fact the natural state of the human body was to be well. Only if the defences were weakened by an imbalance in the personality and the emotions would the agents

The prevention and cure of disease can be found by discovering the wrong within ourselves and eradicating this fault by the earnest development of the virtue which will destroy it; not by fighting the wrong, but by bringing in such a flood of its opposing virtue that it will be swept from our natures.

HEAL THYSELF

ever gain a foothold. This is why he called imbalances the *true* cause of disease.

It follows from this that the best time to take a remedy is when an imbalance first shows itself, long before a physical illness begins. And by the same token if the physical illness is already in place it can be helpful to attack the external agent with a symptom-based medicine or therapy while *at the same time* taking the remedies to regain emotional equilibrium and help restore the body's natural state of wellness.

Treatment bottles

Treatment bottles are the most economical way of taking the remedies, and also the most convenient if you are treating a chronic problem. Try this:

1. Add 2 drops of each selected remedy to a clean 30ml dropper bottle

2. Top up the bottle with still mineral water

3. Take 4 drops from the bottle, 4 times a day, taking the first dose first thing in the morning, the last dose last thing at night and the other two at regular intervals in between

ACCIDENT AND INJURY

Some conditions are purely physical. Suppose, for example, that you are standing on a street corner and a man loses control of his car and runs you over. The cause of your problem is external and has nothing to do with your state of mind, and it is no surprise that orthodox medicine is particularly well equipped to deal with this event.

What the remedies do in such instances is to help us cope with the emotions aroused by the event. They complement orthodox treatment by restoring our good spirits. We can bear the illness with more fortitude and make a quicker recovery.

How many remedies?

Why not put all 38 remedies into a single treatment bottle and cure everything? Dr Bach was asked this question, so he tried it and found that it simply didn't work. It seems that if you take more remedies than you actually need then the ones you don't need will prevent the others from working so effectively.

In practice you will rarely need to give more than six or seven remedies together. Dr Bach gave nine on at least two occasions – but that was in the course of helping thousands of people over a period of years.

TAKING THE REMEDIES

To take the remedies, either drop them on the tongue or take in a teaspoon of water or add to any drink that you would normally have. In a crisis, take additional doses of 4 drops more frequently as required: you can't overdose or build up dependence.

All about dropper bottles

- The dropper bottles you buy do not arrive sterile – but they should be clean enough to use at once, without your having to sterilise them first. If they aren't, get your money back from the shop and go somewhere else.

- If you are halfway through a treatment bottle and decide you need another remedy in addition to the ones you are already taking, simply add 2 drops of the new remedy to the existing mixture. Don't add more water as you will no longer get the minimum dose of the original remedies.

- If you are halfway through a treatment bottle and decide you need other remedies instead of the ones you are already taking, discard the mixture, boil

HYGIENE

If you are putting the drops straight in your mouth be careful not to let the dropper touch your tongue or teeth, as this may contaminate the water in the treatment bottle and make it go off.

Kept in the refrigerator a treatment bottle will last from 2 to 3 weeks, by which time you will need to make up a new one as the water will begin to go stale. If you can't keep your bottle in the fridge you might like to add a teaspoonful of brandy to it as this will help to preserve the water.

Science is tending to show that life is harmony — a state of being in tune — and that disease is discord.
THE ORIGINAL WRITINGS

the bottle up in a saucepan of water to sterilise it and start again.

- If you have finished the contents of a treatment bottle and want to make up the same or a different mix, boil the bottle up in a saucepan of water to sterilise it before you make up the new mixture.

- When boiling dropper bottles, don't boil the rubber teat — there's no need to as the liquid never goes that far up the tube, and rubber doesn't take kindly to being boiled. The glass pipette itself can be removed and boiled along with the bottle, and the screw cap washed separately.

OBTAINING DROPPER BOTTLES

Some large chemists stock 30ml dropper bottles, others stock different-sized dropper bottles, and others don't stock them at all. You can use any size smaller than 30ml, of course, and if you add the same 2 drops of each selected remedy to it you will be sure of getting the minimum dose. But anyone who can sell you Bach Flower Remedies should be able to order standard 30ml dropper bottles for you from the same source, so insist if you don't get what you want first time!

— CASE HISTORY —

Louisa is an unmarried teenager living at home and preparing for her GCSE's. Her period is over a month late. She is terrified of going to the doctor or taking a home pregnancy test in case she is pregnant. None of her friends — including her boyfriend — knows anything is wrong, because she is laughing and joking the same as always. If anything she seems more extrovert than usual. But at night she can't sleep and her work is beginning to suffer.

- Mimulus for the fear of going to the doctor and of being pregnant.

- Agrimony for the mental torment hidden from the world behind a smile.

To bring a patient back from 'not quite himself' to 'quite himself' effects the cure.

QUOTED BY NORA WEEKS,
THE MEDICAL DISCOVERIES OF EDWARD BACH, PHYSICIAN

Hands-on

Pages 37 and 38 are marked out as a diary. This is what to do:

1. Pick a day when you have a few different things to do, such as a meeting to attend, a social event in the evening, a family get-together and so on. As you go through the day try to identify the different moods you go through and write them in the Mood column next to the time. Describe them using any words that make sense to you.

2. At the end of your day – or whenever you next pick up this book – try to identify the remedies you could have used for each of the moods you were in on your Mood Day. Use the list in the Appendix to help you. Write the remedies you select into the Remedy column.

3. Look at the words you used to describe your moods. Are there any cases where the description of the mood as you wrote it doesn't automatically lead to the remedy or remedies that you eventually chose?

– CASE HISTORY –

Colin's behaviour is driving his wife mad. He can't leave the house without turning the gas and electricity off at the mains, and even after doing that he has to check every light switch and gas ring individually. Sometimes he locks the house behind him, then has to unlock it to go and do another check. He knows himself that his behaviour is unusual, but he can't really stop himself.

- Crab Apple for the obsessive over-concentration on minor details.

Today's Date: _____

Time	Mood	Remedy
08.00		
09.00		
10.00		
11.00		
12.00		
13.00		
14.00		

15.00	16.00	17.00	18.00	19.00	20.00	21.00	22.00	23.00

Quick quiz

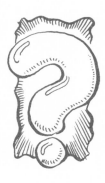

The answers follow immediately after the quiz.

1. How many Bach Flower Remedies are there?

2. Which Bach Flower Remedy would you take to cure a cold?

3. What remedy would you take if you were unnecessarily anxious about your son's welfare?

4. How many drops do you need to take from a stock bottle?

5. What is the difference between the Aspen and Mimulus types of fear?

6. Why did Dr Bach turn away from conventional medicine?

7. Why is Cherry Plum classed as a remedy against fear?

8. What is Rock Rose for?

9. When adding drops to a glass of water, how big a glass should you use?

10. Will a remedy work faster if you drink a whole stock bottle in one go?

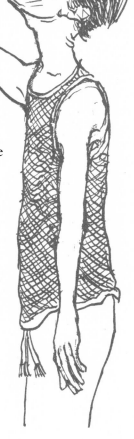

Answers to the quick quiz:

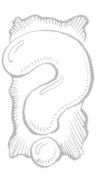

1.   38.

2.   There is no Bach Flower Remedy for colds, or for any other specific physical problem. Instead you would look at the way the cold makes you feel, and use those emotions to start selecting remedies.

3.   Red Chestnut.

4.   Two drops in water, or added to a treatment bottle.

5.   Mimulus is for an ordinary, everyday fear caused by something that you can name. Aspen is for fears with no apparent cause.

6.   Because he wanted to find a way of treating people as individuals rather than simply dealing with their symptoms.

7.   Because if you stop and imagine for a moment that you might lose your self-control and injure yourself or someone else you will see at once that this is a *fearful* thought.

8.   Rock Rose is used for terror and extreme fright.

9.   It doesn't really matter how big the glass is – a small tumbler is ideal.

10. No. As long as the minimum dose is taken (4 drops from a treatment bottle) the full effect is obtained – taking a 'stronger' mix doesn't have a stronger or faster effect.

Day 2

EVERYDAY EMERGENCIES

Let not the simplicity of this method deter you from its use, for you will find the further your researches advance, the greater you will realise the simplicity of all Creation.

QUOTED BY NORA WEEKS,
THE MEDICAL DISCOVERIES OF EDWARD BACH, PHYSICIAN

Rescue Remedy

Rescue Remedy is probably the best known of the Bach Flower Remedies — although in fact it isn't a remedy at all, but a mix of five remedies specially formulated by Dr Bach to deal with the immediate effects of sudden crises and emergencies. The five remedies in Rescue Remedy are:

- Star of Bethlehem for shock.

- Rock Rose for terror and panic.

- Clematis for faintness.

- Impatiens for undue agitation.

- Cherry Plum for loss of self-control and hysteria.

To take Rescue Remedy, put 4 drops in a glass of water and sip at intervals. If there's no water to hand you can put 4 drops straight on the tongue.

Rescue Remedy can be thought of as a first-aid kit — a way of getting through the immediate effects of a crisis. It isn't a cure-all, however, and if you find yourself reaching for the Rescue Remedy too often you might take this as a hint that you need to look at *why* you are always in crisis. Doing this will help you identify the individual remedies that you need for a longer-term solution.

Having said this, there are occasions when a person does in fact need the emergency remedy on a long-term basis. Dr Bach found that where this was the case the Rescue Remedy could be counted as a single remedy for the purpose of making up a treatment — although where you would add 2 drops of individual remedies to a treatment bottle you need to add *4* of Rescue Remedy.

TREATMENT BOTTLES

Just to remind you, a treatment bottle is a 30 ml dropper bottle containing a mix of remedies diluted in water. You take 4 drops from it 4 times a day. See Day 1 for more details.

> *It is only when we attempt to control and rule someone else that we are selfish.*
>
> THE ORIGINAL WRITINGS

Rescue Remedy can be given externally as well as internally, for example if someone is unconscious and so unable to swallow the drops in the normal way. To apply externally, either dab a few drops onto the pulse points or use the diluted remedy to moisten the person's lips.

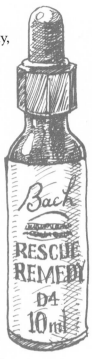

Rescue Cream

Rescue Cream is a lanolin-free cream that contains the same five remedies as Rescue Remedy plus Crab Apple for its cleansing qualities. It is ideal for use on bumps, bruises, cuts and minor burns.

Exercise 2a

Rescue Remedy contains five different remedies, but there is somewhat less of each individual remedy than there would be in a normal, individual stock bottle. Because of this the dosage is doubled, and wherever 2 drops of a single stock bottle would be used you should use 4 drops of Rescue Remedy.

Keeping this in mind, answer TRUE or FALSE to the following statements:

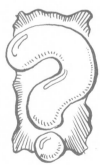

1. In making up a treatment bottle to contain Red Chestnut, Mimulus and Rescue Remedy, you would put 2 drops each of Red Chestnut and Mimulus in the bottle and 4 drops of the Rescue Remedy. TRUE/FALSE

2. For a sudden emergency, simply put 4 drops of the Rescue Remedy in a glass and sip until relief is obtained. TRUE/FALSE

3. If there is no water handy you can put the drops straight on your tongue. TRUE/FALSE

Answers to exercise 2a

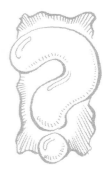

1. TRUE: wherever 2 drops of a single stock bottle would be used you should use 4 drops of Rescue Remedy.

2. TRUE.

3. TRUE.

Remedies for uncertainty

SCLERANTHUS

- 'I want to settle down and raise a family. But I can't make up my mind whether to say yes to Bill's proposal or stop seeing him and hope things work out with George.'

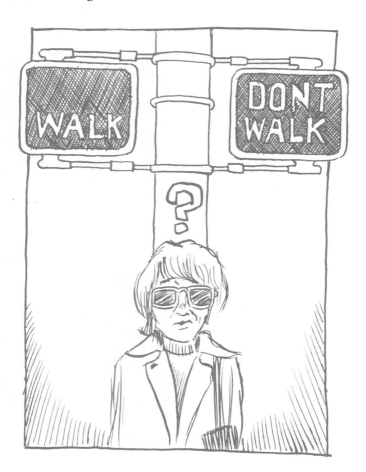

- 'Shopping has become a nightmare. I stand there like an idiot and can't make up my mind about anything.'

Health is our heritage, our right.

THE ORIGINAL WRITINGS

Scleranthus is the remedy for indecision when faced with alternative courses of action.

For example, suppose you are going into town. Should you take the car and risk the traffic and the problem of finding somewhere to park? Or should you take the bus even though this means you might have to wait half an hour at the bus stop and then face the difficulty of getting your bags and packages on board for the return trip? First one answer seems correct, then the other: this is the Scleranthus state.

As this example suggests the Scleranthus uncertainty is often experienced over very trivial matters. Where more important choices are at stake the way to recognise the Scleranthus person is that she will feel indecisive not so much about what she wants from her life, but about how to get it.

The Scleranthus state is a debilitating one since so much energy is used up without anything being achieved. The remedy aims to remove the clouds of uncertainty so that the person can take decisions in a purposeful way and move on.

WILD OAT

- 'I don't know what I want to do, but I don't want to do this.'

- 'I can't see how anything I'm doing here is going to make a difference to anything.'

- 'I've packed the job in and I'm going abroad. I haven't planned anything definite, but maybe things will be different somewhere else.'

Wild Oat people are often very talented and eager to do something really worthwhile with their lives. But they are unable to make up their minds where they want to go, and the result is that all too often they drift from one unsatisfactory situation to another, and fail to advance very much in any particular direction.

If you find it difficult to differentiate between the Scleranthus and Wild Oat states, there are two things to look for. First of all, Scleranthus people find decisions of all types difficult to make, whereas Wild Oat people are usually able to make minor decisions without any problem. Second, Scleranthus people usually have a fairly good idea where they want to be but can't decide how to get there. Wild Oat people on the other hand are often very decisive when faced with alternative courses of action, but the decisions they make may not be productive because

Every one of us is a healer, because every one of us at heart has a love for something.

THE ORIGINAL WRITINGS

they do not have a clear goal in mind. This leaves them feeling dissatisfied and unfulfilled.

Wild Oat helps people in this state to see more clearly what it is that they really want out of life. This allows them to make meaningful changes with some idea of what they want the changes to achieve.

CERATO

- 'I think I might do this – but what do you think?'

- 'What would you do if you were me?'

Cerato people have no trouble making up their mind, but once they have done so they begin to doubt the correctness of their decisions. They then start to go around asking all their friends and acquaintances what they ought to do. They listen to one bit of advice after another and their thoughts are blown in all sorts of different directions. Then when they do act it is often in a different way from

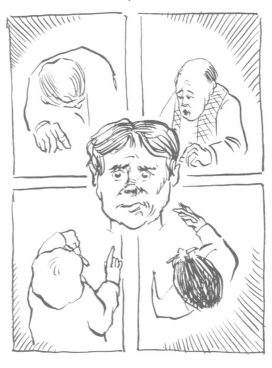

We can judge our health by our happiness.

THE ORIGINAL WRITINGS

the way they first decided on, and they find (too late, and just as they suspected in their hearts) that they should have acted on their first decision after all.

The Cerato remedy is given to increase the person's confidence in his own decisions so that he can take proper charge of his own life, without having to refer to the opinions of others.

HORNBEAM

- 'I wake up in the morning more tired than when I went to bed.'

- 'It takes me ages to get going in the morning because I just can't seem to work up any enthusiasm for the job.'

- 'I feel tired just thinking about it.'

Hornbeam is often called the remedy for the Monday-morning feeling or for the morning after. The Hornbeam lethargy has an emotional cause since no physical or mental effort in the past has caused it — and it can be usefully compared with the Olive remedy, which is for tiredness which comes after doing something. Hornbeam helps lift the spirits so that the task can be taken up, and once the person has managed to do this she often finds that all feelings of exhaustion quickly fade.

GENTIAN

- 'Failed my driving test! That's the end of that, then.'

- 'I was sure I'd get that job. I don't see what I'm going to do now.'

- 'The diet worked at first, but last week I didn't lose anything. I might as well give up.'

Gentian is the remedy for despondency brought on by a setback.

The aim of taking the remedy is to turn this negative defeatism around so that the person is able to get over the setback and either try again or find another way round the obstacle.

GORSE

- 'My sister said you might be able to recommend some of these remedies for me. There's no point, of course — nothing gets rid of these headaches. I'm only here to please her.'

- 'I've tried for eighty jobs and I haven't even had an interview. There's no point applying for any more – it's just a waste of time and money.'

The Gorse state can be seen as a more pronounced version of the Gentian state. The Gorse person doesn't just feel like giving up: he really has given up. He doesn't believe there are any more avenues to explore, even when new possibilities lie right under his nose.

Gorse has been described as 'sunshine in a bottle'. This is partly a tribute to the flower the remedy is made from, which is a deep and radiant yellow, but it is also a reflection of the remedy's positive effects. Gorse shines light back into life so that the dark hopelessness of the Gorse state is replaced with life and light and a renewed determination to take action to make things better.

Exercise 2b

Your friend Helen has a lot of other friends. You have never met them. From her descriptions of their states of mind which remedies do you think they ought to take? You can choose as many as you like from Scleranthus, Cerato, Wild Oat, Hornbeam, Gentian, Gorse – and Rescue Remedy.

1. Bogged down by routine and a dull job, Bob finds it hard to motivate himself in the morning. He wishes he could find a more worthwhile job but doesn't know what sort of career he should consider.

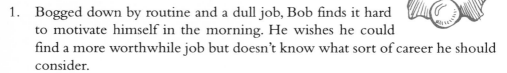

– CASE HISTORY –

Having been kept awake for three nights in a row by his noisy neighbours, Harry loses control when their car alarm starts up at three in the morning and no-one comes to turn it off. He goes out into the street and smashes all the windows and lights on their car. He is burning to get his own back, but at the same time he's scared by the extent of his own rage.

- Cherry Plum for the loss of self-control.

- Holly for the vengeful, spiteful feelings.

There is a factor which science is unable to explain on physical grounds, and this is why some people become afflicted by disease while others escape, although both classes may be open to the same possibility of infection.

HEAL THYSELF

2. Janet has been getting terrible panic attacks. She's gone to the doctor a few times but says she won't be going any more because nothing has done her any good. She says she'll just have to learn to live with it.

3. Harry has been trying to get a job in computing for years. Now he's been offered one. Inside he wants it, but it's a responsible position and he's having trouble saying yes. He's asked me a thousand times what he should do. If he doesn't get a move on they'll give it to someone else.

4. Ronnie was enjoying university until the first time he had to take a seminar. He got a rough ride from the lecturer and it's left him a bit down. He's convinced himself that he'll be a bag of nerves the next time.

5. Fiona can't make up her mind about anything. Going shopping with her is a nightmare – she can spend ten minutes dithering over which loaf of bread to get.

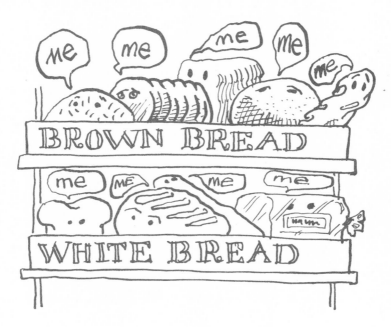

Answers to exercise 2b

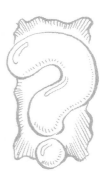

1. Bob could use Hornbeam for his lethargy at the thought of going to his present job, and Wild Oat would help him to decide which direction he should be moving in.

2. Janet would find Rescue Remedy useful for when the panic attacks strike. She could also use Gorse to get her out of her negative hopelessness. This would be preferred to Gentian, since her state is more serious than simple despondency – she really has given up.

3. Harry would need Cerato. Wild Oat isn't appropriate because he knows what career he wants, and neither is Scleranthus because in his heart Harry has made a decision – he just lacks confidence in his judgement.

4. Ronnie has suffered a setback and has let it get to him: Gentian is the correct remedy to select for this. He might also find a bottle of Rescue Remedy handy for the next seminar he has to give, just in case his prediction comes true and he does work himself up into a state.

5. Fiona sounds like a classic Scleranthus person.

The discovery of the remedies

Even when he was working with orthodox and homoeopathic medicines, Dr Bach always trusted his intuition to guide him when other methods failed. And it was his intuition that told him that he would find the new, purer medicine that he was looking for in nature rather than in his laboratory.

– CASE HISTORY –

Having dropped out of university in his final year, and having tried a succession of jobs, none of which were right for him, James is now working for a car importer and feeling, at 30, that his life has been wasted. If only he could find something worth doing…

- Wild Oat to help him see his path in life more clearly.

NARROWING THE SEARCH

Dr Bach felt intuitively that there were some plants that would *not* form part of the new system of medicine that he was perfecting. Nothing poisonous would be used, since he was looking for an entirely gentle method of healing. He would not use food-producing plants, and he would not consider exotic plants such as orchids or those that were too primitive.

The first two of the 38 flower remedies were discovered in Wales in 1928: Impatiens and Mimulus. Later that same year Bach added Clematis to the first two, and the results he achieved with his patients were so remarkable that by the end of the year he had abandoned all other forms of treatment.

Over the next few years Bach wandered all over the English and Welsh countryside. He was extremely sensitive and acutely aware of the healing effects of different plants, and this plus a careful process of trial and error allowed him to find the very few plants that possessed the qualities he was looking for.

By the time he came to Mount Vernon in April 1934 Bach had found 19 remedies. But there was more work to do, and by the spring of the following year his extraordinary sensitivity led to a dramatic outburst of activity. But this stage in his life was also one of great suffering, as Nora Weeks recounts in her book *The Medical Discoveries of Edward Bach, Physician*:

> For some days before the discovery of each one he suffered himself from the state of mind for which that particular remedy was required, and suffered it to such an intensified degree that those with him marvelled that it was possible for a human being to suffer so and retain his sanity; and not only did he pass through terrible mental agonies, but certain states of mind were accompanied by a physical malady in its most severe form.

Between March and August 1935 Dr Bach discovered all of the remaining 19 remedies he needed. Just over a year before he was to die, he announced that his work was complete and that he had achieved what he had set out to do.

To struggle against a fault increases is power, keeps our attention riveted on its presence, and brings us a battle indeed ... To forget the failing and consciously to strive to develop the virtue which would make the former impossible, this is true victory.

HEAL THYSELF

Exercise 2c

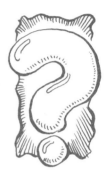

You are talking on the telephone to your friend Robert, who is an expert in the art of selecting remedies. Tell him about the things that have happened to you today – and about how you feel about them. But how do you feel about them? You can work that out by looking at the remedies he selects for you!

YOU:	Hello, Robert
ROBERT:	Hello! What have you been up to?
YOU:	Shopping mainly. I had to get some new clothes.
ROBERT:	That sounds like fun.
YOU:	... (*tell him what happened*)
ROBERT:	Typical Scleranthus! But what do you need a new outfit for?
YOU:	I'm going to John's retirement party on Saturday – and I'm giving the main speech ... (*tell him how you feel about this*)
ROBERT:	Make sure you take some Mimulus if that's how you feel. And carry a bottle of Rescue Remedy with you when you go.
YOU:	I haven't even written the speech yet. Just thinking about putting pen to paper ... (*tell Robert how the thought of writing the speech make you feel*)
ROBERT:	Two drops of Hornbeam added to the mixture!
YOU:	And then there's John himself. I keep worrying ... (*tell him what worries you about John's retiring*)
ROBERT:	That sounds like a job for Red Chestnut. But what about you? Have you decided about buying that house yet?

YOU: Sort of, but … (*tell him how things stand with this decision*)

ROBERT: Well the only advice I'd give is to take some Cerato, forget what other people would do and do what *you* want to do. Anyway, I've got no time to talk now, I've only got 20 minutes to get to the airport before my plane takes off.

YOU: Don't forget the Impatiens!

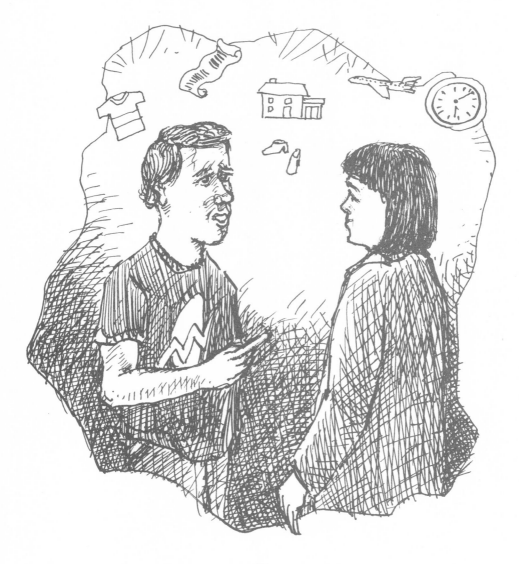

Answers to exercise 2c

You could have described the way you felt and the things that happened using any number of different words, of course, so this is just one of many possible correct answers:

YOU:	Hello, Robert
ROBERT:	Hello! What have you been up to?
YOU:	Shopping mainly. I had to get some new clothes.
ROBERT:	That sounds like fun.
YOU:	No, it wasn't. I couldn't make up my mind whether to get a new suit or something more casual.
ROBERT:	Typical Scleranthus! But what do you need a new outfit for?
YOU:	I'm going to John's retirement party on Saturday – and I'm giving the main speech. Just thinking about speaking in public makes me anxious, and I don't know how I'm going to cope when the day comes.
ROBERT:	Make sure you take some Mimulus if that's how you feel. And carry a bottle of Rescue Remedy with you when you go.
YOU:	I haven't even written the speech yet. Just thinking about putting pen to paper exhausts me. It seems such a lot of work.
ROBERT:	Two drops of Hornbeam added to the mixture!

– CASE HISTORY –

Visiting some friends, Esther picks up a copy of her local paper and learns for the first time that a new motorway is to be built not 200 yards from her quiet country home. She goes pale and has to sit down.

- Star of Bethlehem to help her over the shock.
- Rescue Remedy would be an equally good choice.

... the personality without conflict is immune from illness.
HEAL THYSELF

YOU: And then there's John himself. I keep worrying about whether he'll
            be able to cope with all that leisure time.

ROBERT: That sounds like a job for Red Chestnut. But what about you? Have
            you decided about buying that house yet?

YOU: Sort of, but I'm not sure I'm doing the right thing. George says I
            am, but Dawn says that if she were me ...

ROBERT: Well, the only advice I'd give is to take some Cerato, forget what
            other people would do and do what you want to do. Anyway, I've
            got no time to talk now, I've only got 20 minutes to get to the air-
            port before my plane takes off.

YOU: Don't forget the Impatiens!

Hands-on

Rescue Remedy is a great standby for all kinds of everyday crises and emergencies, from the knot in your stomach when you are late for a meeting to an attack of nerves in the dentist's waiting room. But Rescue Remedy contains five separate remedies, and you don't always need all of them.

For this project, think back to any crises or minor emergencies that you have gone through in the recent past and try to identify five occasions when Rescue Remedy would have been useful. In a few words, jot them down here:

1. ....

    ....

2. ....

    ....

3. ....

....

4. ....

....

5. ....

....

Now imagine that instead of Rescue Remedy you had the five ingredients of Rescue Remedy to hand. Which remedies would you take and which would you leave out? Cross out the ones that do not apply.

1.   Cherry Plum/Clematis/Impatiens/Rock Rose/Star of Bethlehem

2.   Cherry Plum/Clematis/Impatiens/Rock Rose/Star of Bethlehem

3.   Cherry Plum/Clematis/Impatiens/Rock Rose/Star of Bethlehem

4.   Cherry Plum/Clematis/Impatiens/Rock Rose/Star of Bethlehem

5.   Cherry Plum/Clematis/Impatiens/Rock Rose/Star of Bethlehem

Finally, are there any remedies that are not in Rescue Remedy that might have been useful on these occasions? Refer to the list of remedies in the Appendix to help you decide.

Quick quiz

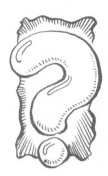

Once again the answers can be found immediately after the quiz.

1. How many individual remedies are there in Rescue Remedy?

2. Which of the Rescue Remedy ingredients is for terror …

3. … and which one is for the fear of losing self-control?

4. When would you use Rescue Cream?

5. What is the sixth ingredient in the Cream and why has it been added?

6. If you can't make up your mind between two possible courses of action, would you need Wild Oat or Scleranthus?

7. What is peculiar about the Hornbeam kind of fatigue?

8. If you were feeling a bit down after something has gone wrong, would you take Gentian or Gorse?

9. In an emergency, how many drops of Rescue Remedy do you take at a time?

10. Is Rescue Remedy stronger if you take it straight from the stock bottle?

— CASE HISTORY —

Julie is very suspicious of her husband. He says he is having to work late because of a new contract his company has just won, but despite the lack of evidence she feels sure that he is seeing someone else, and she is consumed with jealousy. She has been taking her frustrations out on the children, and a couple of times things have got out of control. The strength of her own emotions is beginning to frighten her.

- Holly for the suspicious, jealous thoughts.

- Cherry Plum for the fear that she will lose control of her emotions.

Answers to the quick quiz:

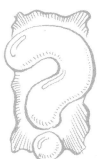

1. Five: Cherry Plum, Clematis, Impatiens, Rock Rose and Star of Bethlehem.

2. Rock Rose.

3. Cherry Plum.

4. You would use Rescue Cream when there was an external trauma that needed calming. Common uses include bruises, swelling, minor burns, wasp stings and grazes.

5. The sixth is Crab Apple, which is added to the cream because of its cleansing qualities.

6. When you know what the alternatives are but hover between them, first one course seeming right and then the other, this is a Scleranthus state. Wild Oat is for the uncertainty people feel when they want to do something worthwhile in their lives but cannot decide what that something should be – in other words, the alternatives themselves are not clear.

7. The Hornbeam fatigue comes at the thought of doing something, in other words before any physical or mental activity has taken place.

8. You would take Gentian for feelings of despondency at a setback. Gorse is for people who lack hope and have given up looking for solutions to the thing that is making them feel depressed.

9. You take 4 drops at a time, ideally by diluting them in a glass of water and sipping from the glass. If there is no water handy you can also put the 4 drops straight on your tongue.

10 It tastes stronger because of the brandy in the stock bottle, but it is just as effective if diluted in water.

Day 3

Type

Remedies

The theory of types

All of the 38 Bach Flower Remedies can be used for moods, and all of us can from time to time fall into these moods. Because of this any one person may need all of the 38 remedies at different times.

Dr Bach also described some of the remedies as *type* remedies, in other words they were linked to basic character types. For example, anyone who was getting impatient would be treated with Impatiens, but in addition there were people who always seemed to be in a hurry and all their lives tended to find the slowness of other people a great trial. For these people Impatiens would be a type remedy, used not for a particular mood ('I feel impatient today') but to correct a fundamental imbalance in the personality ('I'm always impatient').

It's easy to get too wrapped up in trying to define which remedies can be type remedies and which are only ever mood remedies, and as in all

TYPE AND MOOD ASPECTS

As the example of Impatiens shows there is in most cases a direct link between the mood and type side of the type remedies. In other cases the link is not quite so obvious. For example, Mimulus is the remedy for the fear of known things – this is its mood remedy aspect since people of all types can be anxious about things. As a type remedy, it is for people who have always been shy and timid and for this reason may become anxious about crowds and social occasions and so on. The relationship between the type and mood aspects is more subtle in this case, but it is there nevertheless.

– CASE HISTORY –

Told that he is to be made redundant in three month's time, 62-year-old Derek has written hundreds of letters, determined to find another job. So far he hasn't had a single positive answer, but he goes on remorselessly. His wife wishes he would accept that he might have to retire early, but he simply refuses to contemplate defeat, even though he knows himself that his health is beginning to suffer under the strain.

- Oak to help restore his strength and teach him when to fight and when to accept the things he cannot change.

To find the herb that will help us we must find the object of our life.

THE ORIGINAL WRITINGS

things Dr Bach's injunction to keep things simple is the best guide. So don't worry too much at this stage — practice will make perfect, and you'll get opportunities to practise in the rest of this book.

Exercise 3a

Think about the following statements and answer true or false to each one. When you have finished you can check your answers in the following section.

1. Any of the 38 remedies can be type remedies.

    TRUE/FALSE

2. There is no such thing as a Gorse type.

    TRUE/FALSE

3. People can change their type several times in a year.

    TRUE/FALSE

4. The only people who ever get in a negative Vine mood are Vine types — other types always react differently.

    TRUE/FALSE

5. Any of the 38 remedies can be mood remedies.

    TRUE/FALSE

Answers to exercise 3a

1.   False. Some of the remedies do not describe character types. For example, it would be hard to imagine a Star of Bethlehem or Olive type, since these are the remedies for shock and for exhaustion respectively.

2.   True. Gorse is for feelings of hopelessness and despair and is not really a description of a type of person.

3.   False. Your type remedy is a description of your basic personality, and as such is part of what you are.

4.   False. Even shy and timid Mimulus people may occasionally fall into a Vine mood, and try to impose their way of doing things regardless of the effect on others.

5.   True. All of the remedies can be used as mood remedies. This is because on one level they all describe ordinary human emotions that all of us feel at one time or another.

Remedies for over-care for welfare of others

VERVAIN

- 'It was the unfairness of it all that got me. I just had to speak out.'

- 'I'll just get these letters written. It's only midnight.'

- 'How can you believe that? Let me tell you the facts ...'

– CASE HISTORY –

Frank feels nothing but contempt for poor people. If they would only pull themselves together and take a little more care they wouldn't be poor. He has a nice house and car and believes everyone can have the same if they'd only stop being so stupid.

- Beech to help him be more tolerant and understanding of other beliefs and different value systems.

Healing must come from within ourselves.
THE ORIGINAL WRITINGS

The caricature Vervain person is the one who is on the go morning, noon and night, involved in causes and campaigning against injustice in all its forms. But on a more mundane level anyone who feels indignant at injustice or brims over with enthusiasm for a task or ideal might benefit on occasion from the calming effect of Vervain.

Vervain is the remedy for *over*-enthusiasm, and it can be hard to see why too much enthusiasm should be a problem. The danger for the Vervain type is that

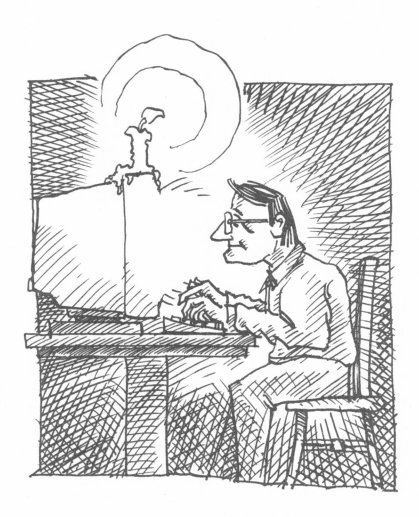

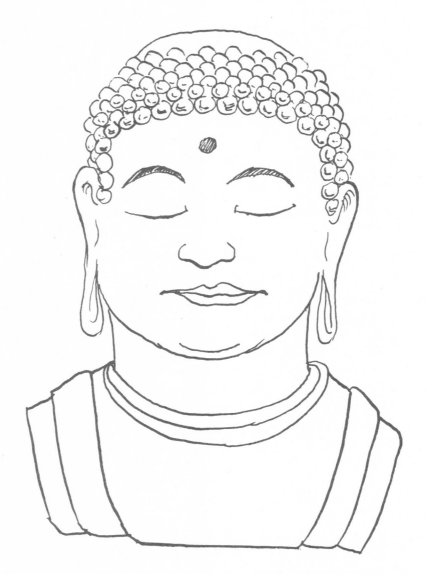

– CASE HISTORY –

Nathan is ten. He is a loving boy, but very possessive, and sulks and cries and screams if he isn't getting his mother's full attention. He's even pretended to be ill so as to get more cuddles.

- Chicory to help him let go and not be so selfish in his love.

her constant mental activity can lead to exhaustion and mental tension. Also, her passion to persuade can turn into fanaticism and an inability to understand other people's points of view. In either case Vervain people can need help to learn how to relax.

Teenagers and recent converts to a cause often fall into negative Vervain moods for a time – as well as becoming a little 'Beechy' ... (see below)

ROCK WATER

- 'I'm sorry, I only ever drink water.'

- 'This is right and that is wrong. I know I'm right, but you can do whatever you want.'

- 'I have made up my mind to run six miles in the morning and in the evening, every day and whatever the weather.'

Where the Vervain uses his energy to try to convert others, the Rock Water person is only concerned with his own salvation. He too has strong opinions, but if he leads at all it is by example only, and he never preaches.

At their negative extreme Rock Water people tend towards martyrdom. This happens when they take their habits of self-denial and self-control to the point where they won't allow themselves pleasure and take little joy in their lives.

In his positive aspect the Rock Water person's strong convictions and high ideals are wholly good – as long as he does not become too rigid and because of this unable to see truth through any lenses but his own. For people in the negative state the remedy can be used to encourage greater flexibility of mind.

BEECH

- 'What a stupid way of carrying on. What's wrong with these people?'

- 'I wish she wouldn't do that all the time. It drives me mad.'

- 'It's his own fault. I've got no sympathy with him.'

The Vervain person seeks to convert others to her way of life; the Rock Water demonstrates the correct path by example; in her negative aspect the Beech person criticises and condemns.

Beech people can be very intolerant of others. They fail to see why everyone doesn't live like them, and never make any allowance for the difficulties others might be facing. They like to have precision and order, not only in their own lives but also in the lives of those around them. They are driven to distraction by the stupidity of people who persist in seeing things differently.

The remedy is taken to encourage tolerance of others so that Beech people can live and let live, and see positive qualities even in people who choose to follow other paths through life.

VINE

- 'Don't argue, just do it.'

- 'Don't tell me – I'm telling you.'

In their positive aspect Vine people are strong, capable leaders and guides. At their most negative they are tyrants who get their own way by using brute force and ruthless domination. They don't criticise the opinions of other people. They ignore them. They may be cruel, and can lack compassion for the people whose lives they blight.

Of course, this is the extreme. The out-of-balance Vine person is not usually so dramatically tyrannous. And all of us can fall into a Vine mood from time to time, when we seek to get our own way by force rather than persuasion.

The remedy is taken to encourage a more flexible, understanding approach to dealing with others, and to bring out those positive qualities that make Vine people so valuable to humanity.

CHICORY

- 'I've never thought of myself. I've done everything for her. And look how she treats me.'

- 'Don't worry about dinner. I'll come round and cook it for you. I won't be in the way.'

- 'I think sometimes you forget that you've got a mother.'

Chicory people have a lot of love to give – but in their negative aspect this love has become possessive and selfish. They care for their loved ones in an obtrusive way, trying to keep them close at hand and controlling their behaviour through correction and admonishment. They can feel very hurt at the slightest snub and may resort to emotional blackmail. The stereotype Chicory person is the parent who won't let grown-up children live their own lives and complains of being neglected if they don't visit three or four times a week.

The remedy is given to encourage the true generosity in the Chicory person. Love can be given freely with no thought of return and without hampering the freedom of others.

The seven groups

Before he began work on his flower remedies, Dr Bach was for many years a bacteriologist at the Royal London Homoeopathic Hospital. There he discovered seven homoeopathic remedies, known as the *Bach Nosodes,* which are still used to this day.

The choice of which nosode to give was originally governed by laboratory diagnosis of specimens. But Dr Bach found that his results were as good if not better if he ignored his laboratory findings and based his selection on the patient's personality rather than the specific medical problem he was suffering from. He categorised each of the seven nosodes in this way for one of seven basic personality types. These were:

- Fear

- Uncertainty

- Insufficient Interest in Present Circumstances

- Loneliness

- Over-sensitivity to Influences and Ideas

- Despondency or Despair

- Over-care for Welfare of Others

Although the nosodes were selected according to character type they were still aimed at physical disease. When Dr Bach decided that he wanted to be able to treat his patients' personalities and emotions directly he left his work on the nosodes behind and turned to the natural world. So began his search for the flower remedies.

When Dr Bach came to write up his final findings in *The Twelve Healers and Other Remedies* he used the original seven headings to categorise the remedies. This is the origin of the seven categories.

The good news about learning the categories is that you don't need to — it is enough to learn the indications for the 38 individual remedies. Nevertheless, the seven headings can provide a useful insight into certain qualities of the individual remedies, as well as a convenient way of splitting the 38 remedies among the seven chapters in this book.

Exercise 3b

Each of the following five people cares too much. Which out of Vine, Beech, Chicory, Vervain and Rock Water best describes each individual?

1.   Every Sunday she goes to church by herself while the rest of the family stays in bed. Then she comes home and spends several hours cooking a roast dinner, and always lays the table with the best silver.

2.   She insists that all her family go to church, and won't hear of any arguments. There's a rota for cooking Sunday dinner and if it's your turn it's your turn and that's that – but if she is busy when it's her turn she can always get her husband to cook instead.

3.   She's forever criticising her lazy family who can't haul themselves out of bed in time to come to church with her. She comes home and is irritated to discover that her son has peeled the potatoes instead of scrubbing them.

WHY PUT THAT THERE?

It can be interesting to reflect on why Dr Bach placed remedies in a particular category. For example, Gentian is commonly thought of as the remedy for discouragement and mild depression after a setback. Why then does it appear under the 'Uncertainty' heading rather than 'Despondency or Despair'? Perhaps Dr Bach was stressing how the Gentian setback causes a loss of will power and faith – in other words, a loss of certainty. The Gentian state is not true despair because it could be overcome if the person were more certain of his ability to progress.

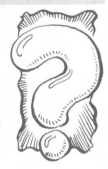

— CASE HISTORY —

Jenny enjoys poetry, classical music and walks in the country, preferably with her dog for company. Since moving to Scotland she has lost contact with her few close friends and is finding it difficult to meet new ones. Even if she could face the hurly-burly of the village pub she might not find it any easier to get to know people, because the locals think she is a bit stuck up.

• Water Violet to help her relax more with other people and seem less aloof.

— CASE HISTORY —

Vera has been suffering from headaches, and they've been getting worse. She won't go to see a doctor because she says it runs in her family: her father and his father both had the same thing, and just as nobody could help them, so nothing can be done for her.

- Gorse to overcome her hopelessness so that she can see a path out of her difficulties and follow it.

4. She tries to persuade her family to come to church with her on Sundays — as she says, it's for their own good. Sunday dinnertime is usually spent arguing about politics, and sometimes the family has to make do with a sandwich if she's got a meeting to go to in the afternoon.

5. She tries to persuade her family to come to church with her on Sundays — as she says, it's one of the few chances they have to go out together as a family. She always cooks a proper roast dinner, of course, and she gets upset if her eldest son can't come home to help eat it — which he can't very often because he's married now and has children of his own.

— CASE HISTORY —

Now in his late thirties, and married with children and a demanding career, Oliver is plagued by thoughts of his teenage years. He remembers first romances, nights out with friends and the boundless energy of being seventeen years old. Everyday life for him now seems flat and drab in comparison and he is having trouble finding things to look forward to.

- Honeysuckle to help him live life in the present, just like he did when he was seventeen.

Answers to exercise 3b

1. Rock Water.

2. Vine.

3. Beech.

4. Vervain.

5. Chicory.

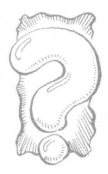

Identifying type remedies

As we have seen some of the Bach Flower Remedies describe types of people. One of them – perhaps a couple, since some people are a bit of a mixture – will describe you. But how do you find out which one, and why do you need to know anyway?

One way of identifying your type remedy is to look at how you tend to react when things are going wrong. If you are a Vine type, for example, you will *usually* react to too much stress at work by attempting to bulldoze your way through and get your own way at the expense of other people. If you are a Mimulus person the same trigger will *probably* cause you to draw back into yourself and your shyness may come to the fore.

The type remedy points, then, to a particular weakness in you. And just as you might carry a packet of throat lozenges around if you tend to get sore throats, so you might well carry a bottle of Beech around if you tend to become intolerant. On a deeper level, type remedies help you to think about who you are and about the particular qualities you need to work at and develop.

It's important, though, not to get too hung up on type remedies. Even the most dyed-in-the-wool Vine will occasionally need Centaury (the remedy for those who find it hard to say 'no' to other people), or any of the other remedies. And sometimes we pretend to be different as a way of coping when things go wrong. A timid child who acts tough to cope with his tough school may get into the habit of acting tough until he forgets that he was ever different. This doesn't really matter, since the remedies will eventually uncover the real person. Treat what you most obviously see in yourself and you will not go far wrong.

Indeed, sometimes the real type remedy is the last thing you find at the end of a long journey of self-discovery. There's no need to worry if you can't see the end of the journey when you are just starting out.

Exercise 3c

For this exercise you will need to know some remedies that haven't been covered in detail yet. Because of this, you might want to start by looking at this list of indications, taken from the Appendix:

AGRIMONY — For mental torment hidden behind a smiling face

CHESTNUT BUD — For repeated errors and the inability to learn from experience

CLEMATIS — For day-dreaming, and living in an idealised future rather than the everyday present

IMPATIENS — For impatience

OAK — For strong people who struggle on past the limits of their strength

VINE — For dominant people who rule others with a rod of iron

WILLOW — For self-pity, resentment and the blaming of others

Now look at the personalities whose names appear below. Which of the remedies listed above would make good type remedies for them? (You may suggest more than one if you want.)

1. Charlie Chaplin as the little tramp.

2. Don Quixote.

3. Donald Duck.

4. Shakespeare's Richard III.

5. Marilyn Monroe.

6. Wile E Coyote (in the Roadrunner cartoons).

Every single person has a life to live, a work to do, a
glorious personality, a wonderful individuality.

THE ORIGINAL WRITINGS

Answers to exercise 3c

1. For Chaplin's tramp you might have considered Agrimony (the smiling face masking inner torture), Oak (plodding on and refusing to give in), or Clematis (a dreamer, living more in fantasy than in reality).

2. Don Quixote was the reader of romantic novels who dreamt of becoming a knight-errant and charged windmills under the impression they were giants. His dreamy nature and lack of interest in the present probably indicate that he would have been a Clematis type.

3. Donald Duck loses his patience at the drop of a hat when things don't go his way. Impatience is probably the trigger for his irritability, so Impatiens would be the obvious choice.

4. His self-pity and bitterness in the first speech of the play ('Now is the winter of our discontent …') might make you think that Shakespeare's Richard III was a Willow type. In fact experience has shown that there are few if any true Willow types (they turn out to be something else under the Willow mood), and Vine would be a better choice for Richard, who is a determined, ruthless tyrant who sticks at nothing to get his way.

5. Even when she was in despair deep down Marilyn Monroe still appeared happy and carefree for the cameras. She could well be a typical Agrimony type.

– CASE HISTORY –

Penelope arrives home from work too exhausted to play with the children.

- Olive to lift her tiredness.

6. Wile E Coyote could probably do with some Chestnut Bud to help him to learn from his repeated failure to catch the Roadrunner – but Chestnut Bud is not usually thought of as a type remedy. Oak would be the obvious choice here, since Wile E Coyote simply refuses to give in, and goes on pursuing his aim in the teeth of every failure.

Hands-on

1. On separate pieces of paper, write out the names of the following remedies: Mimulus, Red Chestnut, Aspen, Rock Rose, Cherry Plum, Scleranthus, Cerato, Wild Oat, Hornbeam, Gentian, Gorse, Vervain, Rock Water, Beech, Vine and Chicory

2. Shuffle the pieces of paper then deal out five remedies at random

3. Try to imagine the character and situation of someone who would need all five remedies and no others

If you are not sure what a remedy is for, look back through the book to check it before you start

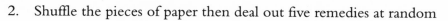

– CASE HISTORY –

After sharing a flat with her for six months, William is becoming more and more irritated by Siobhan's presence. He doesn't like the programmes she watches on TV, the fact that she takes a bath in the evenings or the food she cooks. He wants to give Siobhan a remedy that will make her more like him.

- Beech – for William! – to help him be more tolerant of other people.

The sun and boiling methods

Dr Bach prepared his remedy plants using two simple methods. The sun method involved taking the flower heads from selected plants, floating them in a glass bowl filled with water and leaving them in full sunlight for three hours. The boiling method, which he mainly used for the tougher, woodier plants such as Aspen, Willow and Elm, was a matter of collecting flowers, stems and twigs in a saucepan and boiling them for half an hour.

These two simple methods are still used today by the trustees of Dr Bach's home, Mount Vernon. The prepared remedies are mixed 50/50 with brandy to make the mother tincture. There are approximately two-thirds of a drop of mother tincture – diluted in more brandy – in every single-remedy stock bottle sold.

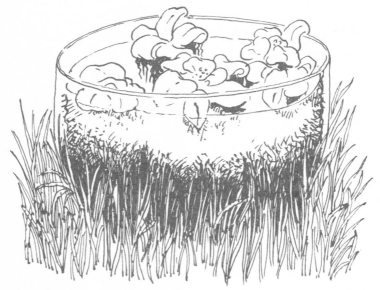

– CASE HISTORY –

Lynne has always been a quiet, shy sort of person. Promotion at work means she should be more assertive now in order to motivate others, but instead she seems even more determined to be invisible, and goes bright red if attention is drawn to her.

- Mimulus to help her overcome her shyness and lose her fear of being noticed.

Exercise 3d

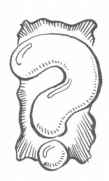

For this exercise, think of six different people who would each need one of the type remedies listed below. You can choose someone you know, a famous person, or a character from literature, television or films. You haven't covered all these remedies yet, so where this is the case brief indications are given to help you.

1. Chicory.

2. Vervain.

3. Water Violet (private people who can appear proud or aloof).

4. Oak (strong people who struggle on past the limits of their strength).

5. Heather (self-obsessed people who talk constantly of their own affairs and need an audience).

6. Centaury (willing servants who find it hard to say 'no').

WORKING IN PAIRS

If you are working through this book with a partner, see if she can guess what remedies the person needs based entirely on your description of his character and situation. Then swap roles and let your partner pick the remedies and create the scenario while you try to guess which remedies were selected.

— CASE HISTORY —

Ruth is in her 80's. She is a strong-minded lady who enjoys giving advice and guidance to others. When she has a fall and is confined to bed she is for the first time dependent on a nurse coming in to cook and take care of her. She misses being in charge, and begins to think that she won't ever be herself again.

- Vine, her type remedy, to help her accept help when she needs it.

- Gorse to overcome the pessimistic hopelessness.

Answers to exercise 3d

Everyone will find different answers to this exercise, but here are some suggestions:

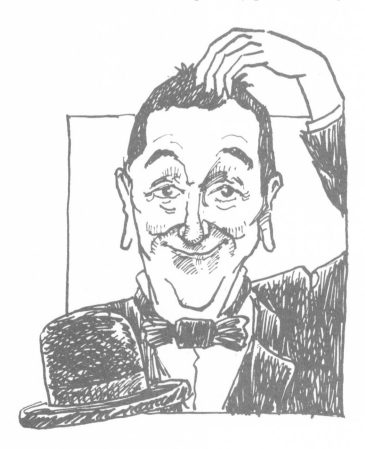

1. Some people might list their mothers or mothers-in-law in this category, but fathers and fathers-in-law can also expect attention in return for love ...

2. Vervain types could include the botanist and environmentalist David Bellamy, the anti-slavery campaigner William Wilberforce, and politicians like Tony Benn and Edwina Currie, who both pursued a cause regardless of the political cost to themselves. Then there is Superman, who fights for truth, justice and the American way ...

3. Water Violet types could include France's rather aloof ex-president, François Mitterrand and PG Wodehouse's perfectly-poised butler Jeeves ...

4.   Oak types could include Winston Churchill, the mythological character Sisyphus, who was condemned to roll a stone up a hill for all eternity, and Douglas Bader, the fighter pilot who had both legs amputated but got straight back into the cockpit as soon as he was released from hospital …

5.   Heather types could include the lonely and unhappy gossip Miss Bates in Jane Austen's *Emma* …

6.   Centaury types could include Stan Laurel out of Laurel and Hardy and Lou Costello out of Abbott and Costello, as well as the everyday victims of negative Vine and Chicory people and of course Cinderella …

Quick quiz

Once more, the answers can be found immediately after the quiz.

1.   How many of the 38 remedies can be used for passing moods and temporary emotional states?

2.   What is a type remedy?

3.   Vervain seems to be entirely positive – committed, enthusiastic, hard-working – so when would a Vervain person need the remedy?

4.   If the Bach Flower Remedies don't treat physical problems directly, how can taking them make you better?

5.   Referring back to the list of type remedies in exercise 3d, which of them might be a good type remedy for Samson, the strong man who refused to give in and pulled the temple down on his own head as that was the only way to defeat his enemies?

6.   Do you have to wait until you are sick to use the remedies?

7.   What is the main difference between the Vervain and Vine types?

8.   Do people change their types over time?

9.   Is it absolutely essential to include your type remedy in every treatment bottle you make for yourself?

10.   Is there such a thing as a Cherry Plum type?

Answers to the quick quiz:

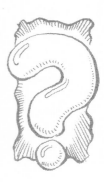

1   All of them.

2. It is a remedy that describes someone's basic nature. We all can get into moods where we want our loved ones around us and feel rejected if we don't get the attention we feel we deserve, but if you always tend to be like this when things go wrong then Chicory is probably your type remedy.

3. Vervain people don't need the remedy because they are enthusiastic, but only when their enthusiasm leads them to extremes. They may take on too much and drive themselves too hard so that their emotional and physical health begins to suffer, or they may become very fixed in their views and incapable of changing their minds.

4. Our emotional states affect our immune system and our body's ability to stay well. Put simply, balanced people don't get sick as much as unbalanced people do. So by balancing negative emotions with the remedies your body is better equipped to take care of itself.

5. Oak might be a good choice, indicated by his strength and refusal to bow to circumstance.

6. No – the most effective way to use them is to make them part of your life, so that you treat minor imbalances before they are able to take root and manifest as physical problems.

7. Vervain people want you to believe the same things they believe. Vine people often don't care what you believe, as long as you do what they think is right. Where Vervain people argue and persuade, Vine people order.

8. If someone seems to have changed types, it is more likely that the real type has been obscured underneath a shell, created perhaps to let the person cope with a difficult time. Because the real type describes basic characteristics, these do not usually change in a single lifetime.

9. In most cases you will probably include your type remedy anyway. But there's no rule that says you have to, so if you don't need it, don't include it.

10. Cherry Plum is for the fear of losing control and doing something terrible either to yourself or to someone else. This is not a description of an innate characteristic, so Cherry Plum is not usually thought of as a type remedy.

Day 4

The
Holistic
Approach

Orthodox, alternative and complementary

Orthodox medicine is a name sometimes given to the technology-rich, interventionist medicine practised in the West. It has had numerous and spectacular triumphs. It is the first therapy to which most of us turn when there is a mechanical fault in our bodies and something stops working properly. But in many cases it confines itself to dealing with symptoms and doesn't try to correct the imbalances that may have caused the mechanical problem to arise in the first place.

Alternative medicine and *Complementary medicine* seek to find a different path to health. Theirs has been termed a *holistic* approach. They address the whole person as well as or instead of the specific physical symptoms.

Many people use the terms alternative and complementary as if they were equivalent. But there is a distinction, and it lies in the way a therapy is used. Those who practise alternative medicine see themselves in opposition to ortho-

TENSION EQUALS VERVAIN?

At one stage of his work Dr Bach thought that there would be a link between particular disorders and particular personality or emotional imbalances. Indeed, in his book *Heal Thyself* he says that 'the very part of the body affected is no accident, but is in accordance with the law of cause and effect'. Some people still act on this belief today, and take Vervain when they feel tense, or select Rock Water for everyone with a stiff neck.

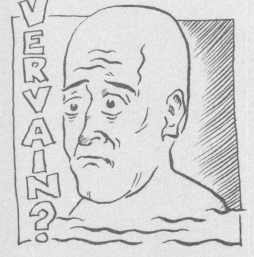

But *Heal Thyself* was published in 1931; by the time Dr Bach had completed his research he knew that in fact the physical disease did not give any clue to selecting the right remedy. Instead, as he said in a lecture in 1936, 'The manner in which a patient reacts to an illness is alone taken into account. Not the illness itself.' (See *The Original Writings of Edward Bach*, edited by Judy Howard and John Ramsell.) All sorts of people can feel tense, but Vervain would only be given to people whose tension was accompanied by over-enthusiasm, a strong sense of injustice or commitment to a cause.

dox medicine. They may advise their patients not to see orthodox doctors and counsel against the use of orthodox medicines.

People practising with the Bach Flower Remedies, on the other hand, usually fall into the complementary school, and see a place for other forms of treatment alongside their own. This is because the remedies can be used in conjunction with any other course of treatment or medicine and will neither interfere with such treatments nor be interfered with by them. No practitioner registered with the Dr Edward Bach Foundation, for example, will ever tell you to stop taking another treatment or advise you to disobey the advice of your GP: there is no need to.

In any case, even if orthodox medicine *is* dealing with symptoms alone that is no reason in itself not to use it. The remedies in Dr Bach's system do not need the physical symptoms in order to start working on the emotional cause, since they take no account of them. In other words: don't ask yourself how you feel, ask *how you feel about the way you feel …*

Exercise 4a

As we have seen, there is no one remedy for gout, M.E., the common cold or any other physical problem. Different people suffering from the same *physical* problem will take different remedies if their *personalities* are different.

Here are three people with the same physical problem. See if you can pick the correct type remedy for each one. (All of the correct remedies have already been described in previous chapters, but you can refer to the Appendix for remedy indications if you want to.)

1. 'I get stomach pains after every meal. I've always been a worrier, I suppose, and it's been much worse since I had children. Even now they're grown up I'm terrified in case something happens to them.'

2. 'I get stomach pains after every meal. I can't make up my mind whether or not to go to the doctor with it. But then I'm just not a very decisive person, I suppose.'

3. 'I get stomach pains after every meal. I don't know why because I'm always very careful about what I eat, and I never drink more than a single glass of wine a day out of principle. My wife says it's because I drive myself too hard, but there it is: I've got standards and I'm not about to let them slip.'

Answers to exercise 4a

1. Red Chestnut.

2. Scleranthus.

3. Rock Water.

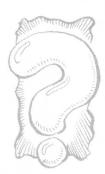

Dealing with physical problems

Dr Bach described the flower remedy system as 'the most perfect which has been given to mankind within living memory' because it was so simple and because it treated the real root cause of disease, i.e. imbalances in the personality itself. This does not mean, however, that the Bach Flower Remedies are the only way of helping you when you have already become sick.

For a start there are medical problems whose cause is entirely external, such as food poisoning and broken bones, and in these cases treatment by the remedies is not to be taken as an alternative to proper orthodox medical attention. The best thing for a broken bone is to set it straight – it is a mechanical problem and demands a mechanical solution.

Then there are cases where an imbalance has gone on so long that a physical problem has already developed. For example, emotional stress might make you susceptible to a virus. While restoring balance will help your body to fight off the invader, other means can be used as well to make sure it is dealt with all the quicker. Remember that the remedies are *complementary* medicines and not *alternatives*.

– CASE HISTORY –

Norma is married to her career at an advertising agency. She doesn't even try to switch off, and weekends are simply a chance to get to work and do some planning while the office is quiet. She's not unhappy – on the contrary she loves what she is doing and is full of enthusiasm – but she has had a few niggling illnesses recently and even her boss has told her to slow down.

- Vervain to curb her over-enthusiasm and bring some balance into her life.

In illness there is a change of mood from that in ordinary life, and those who are observant can notice this change often before, and sometimes long before, the disease appears, and by treatment can prevent the malady ever appearing.

THE TWELVE HEALERS AND OTHER REMEDIES

Certainly all of the people in the last exercise should be seeing a GP, if they haven't already done so, since their symptoms may indicate the presence of a physical problem such as an ulcer. This may need treating in its own right.

Hands-on

You will have to refer to the remedy descriptions in the Appendix to complete this project.

1. Take a notepad, a pencil and a quiet evening, and watch all your favourite television programmes.

2. Try to select type and mood remedies for the characters and personalities who appear.

3. Think about the following general questions:

- How much can you tell about character from the clothes people wear?

- How reliable are facial expressions and body language as guides to mood and personality?

- Were there any characters whose type remedy was obvious at first glance? What made the selection obvious?

- Were there any characters whose emotional state didn't seem to fit into Dr Bach's scheme?

If the answer to the last question is 'yes', try looking for the cause of the emotions you witnessed. There is no one remedy for anger in Dr Bach's system, for example, but several different remedies can apply depending on the cause of the anger. Can the same reasoning apply to the cases you have noted?

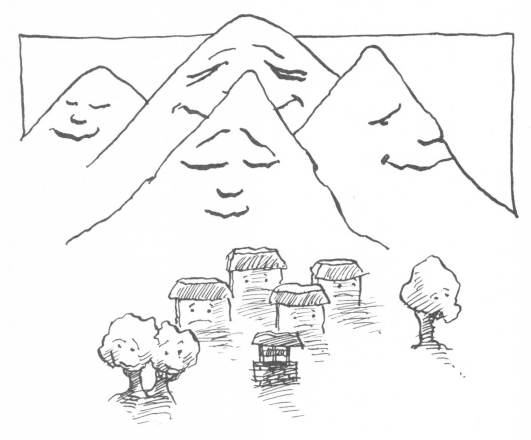

METAPHORS

When you describe something in terms of something else you are using a metaphor. So if you write 'the proud mountains raised their heads far above the timid village' you are describing scenery (mountains and a village) in terms of human emotions (pride and timidity). A metaphor is a useful way of describing something, but it should not be taken literally: neither the mountains nor the village feel pride, timidity or anything else.

How do the remedies work?

Perhaps the hardest thing for people to understand about the Bach Flower Remedies is how flowers can heal emotions. In a sense every attempt to answer this question involves using a metaphor, because in truth we still understand nothing at all about life and consciousness and emotions, except what our metaphors tell us.

The metaphors used change over time, of course. In his earlier writings Dr Bach used the metaphor of vibrations, and spoke of sympathetic vibrations between particular plants and particular

Behind all disease lie our fears, our anxieties, our greed, our likes and dislikes.

THE TWELVE HEALERS AND OTHER REMEDIES

states of mind. Now many people talk of the remedies as 'energy medicines' and believe that, like homoeopathy, they work at the level of energy.

In the final analysis the metaphors used to describe the way the remedies work are not really very important. In fact they can be dispensed with altogether. This is what Dr Bach did: by the time he finished his work and prepared the final edition of *The Twelve Healers* he no longer felt it necessary to talk about vibrations. 'No science, no knowledge is necessary, apart from the simple methods described herein,' he said, dictating the new introduction to *The Twelve Healers* in 1936, 'and they who will obtain the greatest benefit from this God-sent Gift will be those who keep it pure as it is; free from science, free from theories; for everything in Nature is simple.'

Remedies for loneliness

HEATHER

- 'I'm off to the club tonight, well I thought I should go, though I don't really feel like it because of this leg. Did I tell you about my leg? The doctor said he'd never seen anything like it, but it doesn't stop me getting to the shops. I've just been there, just now, as it happens – I needed some tea. I ran out this morning, it always happens when you're in a hurry, and of course I … I … I ….'

> ### – CASE HISTORY –
>
> Dawn has a slight cold. She wraps herself up in blankets, doses herself on cold cures and vitamins, and gets on the phone to all her friends and relations to tell them how awful she feels.
>
> - Heather for the self-absorption and over-concentration on petty ills.

Heather people are wrapped up in their own affairs and problems, so much so that they take no interest in the problems of others. Because they are scared of being lonely they try to turn anyone who comes their way into an audience – but as their incessant talking is tiresome others begin to avoid them so that they end up lonely, just as they feared they would.

The positive effect of the remedy is to help people in the Heather state rise above their own concerns and turn their thoughts out to others. They become better listeners and so are able to share their troubles with others effectively, instead of simply inflicting their problems on whoever crosses their paths. Well-balanced Heather people are a help and support to others.

IMPATIENS

- 'Give it to me, I'll do it.'

- 'I can't stop, I'm in a rush.'

- 'I haven't got all day.'

The Impatiens person is always in a hurry. Usually quick-witted, she has no patience with the slow, methodical people of this world. If she has to wait for someone to do something she becomes tremendously frustrated and irritable. For this reason she usually prefers to work and act alone, so avoiding the need to explain and consult with people whose approach to life is more measured. Look for mannerisms such as drumming fingers, fidgeting, tapping feet and other signs of impatience.

Emotions like these can lead not only to stress and tension but also to accidents caused by rushing into things and trying to do things too quickly. Many an Impatiens person has slammed a finger in a door or tried to carry one too many cups back to the draining board! The remedy restores calm and balance. It teaches patience and the ability to value more methodical souls for the different skills and capabilities they bring to life.

– CASE HISTORY –

Kelly has been offered two jobs. One pays more money; the other looks more exciting. She cannot for the life of her decide which one to accept.

- Scleranthus to help her to stop hesitating and know her own mind.

WATER VIOLET

- 'I'll leave you to get on with this in your own way.'

- 'I prefer my own company.'

- 'You go your way, I'll go mine.'

The Water Violet flower grows on the tip of a long, slender, erect stalk — and the personality associated with it is very similar. Water Violet people are nature's aristocrats: capable, graceful, centred and private. They are happy with their own company and never intrude on the privacy of others. Balanced Water Violet people are a joy to all around them.

The danger for these quiet souls is that their tendency to stay aloof from the rest of struggling humanity can make them appear proud and difficult to know. When they do want some companionship there may not be anyone left willing to give it. They may also get so used to their own company that they find it difficult to develop close relationships. The remedy is used when necessary to help people of this type to open up more to other people so that they don't grow too isolated.

Exercise 4b

You have received some letters from friends who would like your advice. Using your knowledge, give your considered responses.

A. Dear _____

I've had this bad back for about six years now. The doctor says he can't find anything wrong physically, but things have got worse and worse and now I am on more or less permanent sick leave.

What remedies should I take for this problem? My employer has been sympathetic up to now but I am scared that if something can't be done soon I'll lose my job.

Yours

John

THE BACH REMEDIES WORKBOOK

B. Dear _____

I'm a bit confused over dosage. You told me to take Rescue Remedy by putting 4 drops into water and then sipping from the glass, but the man at the shop told me to take 4 drops straight from the bottle 4 times a day. Which is right?

All the best

Yvonne

C. Dear _____

I'd like to know what you think about two of the people at work. They've both been suffering on and off with very bad sinus trouble and I'm not sure what the right remedy is for that. Let me tell you a bit about them.

George has really let the whole thing get to him. He's always been a bit of a chatterbox but over the last few months it's been getting worse, and all he wants to do is moan on and on about the pains in his sinus, and what he did and didn't do to try to sort it out. It's such a pain to listen to that people are starting to avoid him. But the biggest problem I think will be trying to get him to take any remedies because he's managed to convince himself that nothing can do him any good and that he'll just have to suffer the rest of his life. He really is quite depressed.

Jenny is very different. She's just withdrawn into herself and is determined to suffer in silence. People at work think she's stuck up, and it's true that she's always liked her own company, but I think it's got to the point now when she's almost forgotten how to open up to other people and I think that sometimes she feels a bit lonely. She'd never say that, of course.

Any ideas?

Katherine

– CASE HISTORY –

Emily's dream is to be a vet, but she fails crucial examinations in her final year and this leaves her too discouraged to start studying for the re-sit later in the year.

- Gentian to help her over this setback and give her encouragement to start work again.

Answers to exercise 4b

Here are some (suggested) model replies. How did you match up? Maybe you did better — but if your answers are markedly different from these, take some time to think about why.

A. Dear John

There isn't a single remedy for bad backs because the remedies don't treat physical complaints directly. What they can do is correct any emotional imbalances you may have so that your body will be better able to regain its health naturally.

Why don't you pop round for a chat? We could talk a bit about you and how you feel at the moment. Armed with this information I'll be able to suggest some remedies for you to consider.

In the meantime, there is one remedy you could start taking right away, and that is Mimulus. That is the remedy for known, everyday fears: in this case the fear that you might lose your job. I'm sure that this fear is not helping you get better quickly, so you would be better off without it.

Yours

———

B. Dear Yvonne

We're both right, in a way. If you are taking Rescue Remedy because you are going through a crisis of some kind (which is the normal reason to take it), then you are right to put 4 drops in water and sip from the glass. Of course, if there is no water handy you can take the 4 drops straight on your tongue, and repeat as needed.

The man in the shop is also right, in that if you are treating a long-term condition (for example, if you are suffering frequent panic attacks) then you need to take the doses regularly. In this case you could indeed take 4 drops four times a day from your stock bottle. But a more economical method would be to make up a treatment bottle by adding 4 drops of Rescue Remedy to a 30ml dropper bottle and then topping this up with still mineral water. Then take 4 drops four times a day from *this* bottle. You are using much less remedy but you will get the same effect. (And you can of course take additional drops as and when you need them.)

Yours

———

C. Dear Katherine

There is no one remedy for sinus trouble, or any other physical condition. Instead Dr Bach said that the correct way to select remedies was to ignore the physical problem and look at the individual's personality and emotions. Fortunately you have told me enough for me to suggest some remedies for your two friends.

For George, I would suggest Heather and Gorse. George sounds like a person who likes the company of others, but he might be having trouble understanding that he has to give attention as well as take it. The Heather is to help him to look beyond his own troubles so that he can think more about others. The Gorse should help overcome the rather forlorn, hopeless feeling he has at the moment, so that he can start exploring new ways forward in a more optimistic frame of mind.

As for Jenny, she sounds like a typical Water Violet person, and this is the remedy I would suggest to help her to relax and unbend a little so that she won't have to suffer alone.

Let me know how they both get on.

Yours

———

Emotions and health

Dr Bach believed there was a direct link between emotions and health. 'Disease is a kind of consolidation of a mental attitude,' he wrote to a colleague in 1930. And indeed everyday life is full of examples of how thoughts, feelings and beliefs can have a direct physical consequence.

Orthodox medicine has been rediscovering this truth for itself over the last twenty years. Most doctors now accept that people who approach their illnesses in a positive way get better more quickly. The old saying 'laughter is the best medicine' has proved to be correct as well: it seems that the immune system is capable of picking up information from the central nervous system, and that unhappiness impedes the body's defences just as happiness helps it.

Dr Bach would not have been surprised at this change in attitudes. He always spoke of his system as the medicine of the future. It seems that today the future is almost upon us.

Nothing in nature can hurt us when we are happy and in harmony, on the contrary all nature is there for our use and our enjoyment

THE ORIGINAL WRITINGS

Exercise 4c

Look at the story below and cross out the remedy choices that do *not* apply.

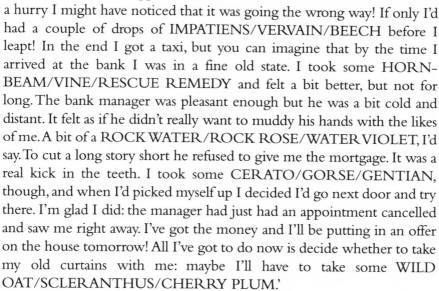

'I had a real day of it yesterday. I'd just left the house when I ran into Ethel, and of course it was twenty minutes before I could escape. She's a real MIMULUS/HEATHER/RED CHESTNUT, that one. When I did manage to get away I was already late so I hopped on a bus. If I hadn't been in such a hurry I might have noticed that it was going the wrong way! If only I'd had a couple of drops of IMPATIENS/VERVAIN/BEECH before I leapt! In the end I got a taxi, but you can imagine that by the time I arrived at the bank I was in a fine old state. I took some HORN-BEAM/VINE/RESCUE REMEDY and felt a bit better, but not for long. The bank manager was pleasant enough but he was a bit cold and distant. It felt as if he didn't really want to muddy his hands with the likes of me. A bit of a ROCK WATER/ROCK ROSE/WATER VIOLET, I'd say. To cut a long story short he refused to give me the mortgage. It was a real kick in the teeth. I took some CERATO/GORSE/GENTIAN, though, and when I'd picked myself up I decided I'd go next door and try there. I'm glad I did: the manager had just had an appointment cancelled and saw me right away. I've got the money and I'll be putting in an offer on the house tomorrow! All I've got to do now is decide whether to take my old curtains with me: maybe I'll have to take some WILD OAT/SCLERANTHUS/CHERRY PLUM.'

Answers to exercise 4c

Heather, Impatiens, Rescue Remedy, Water Violet, Gentian, Scleranthus.

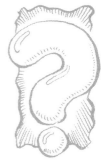

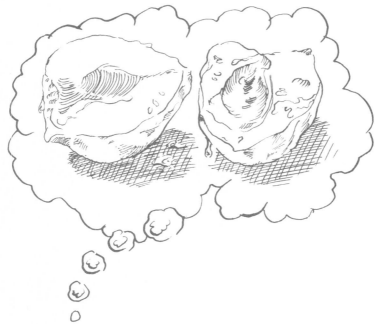

AN EXPERIMENT

If you don't believe that your state of mind has a direct effect on your body, try this simple experiment:

- Close your eyes and imagine a ripe, juicy peach, cut in half and lying on a plate

- Now imagine picking up one of the halves of peach and biting into it. Imagine the feel of the furry skin on your tongue, then the feel of the flesh as you bite into it and the juice rolling down your chin

- Now concentrate on the slightly sharp, sweet taste of the peach juice and then think about chewing and swallowing the fruit and its juice

You have just produced an increase in the rate of saliva flow – a physical change – simply by thinking about something!

As the herbs heal our fears, our anxieties, our worries, our faults and our failings, it is these we must seek, and then the disease, no matter what it is, will leave us.

THE TWELVE HEALERS AND OTHER REMEDIES

Quick quiz

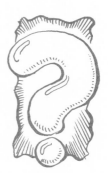

Once more the answers can be found immediately after the quiz.

1. Can you take the Bach Flower Remedies at the same time as other medicines?

2. Are there any physical symptoms that provide clues about which remedy to select?

3. Why did Dr Bach believe that the remedies he had discovered would be valid for all time?

4. What are the indications for Water Violet?

5. Dr Bach grouped Heather, Impatiens and Water Violet under the heading 'loneliness'. Does this mean that everyone who feels lonely needs at least one of these remedies?

6. Heather and Water Violet people are opposites – in what way?

7. What positive quality does Impatiens represent?

8. Impatiens and Beech people can both be irritated by others. What's the difference between them?

9. What is Cerato for?

10. If you wanted to be more self-reliant and be able to enjoy being alone, would you take Water Violet?

THE BACH REMEDIES WORKBOOK

Answers to the quick quiz:

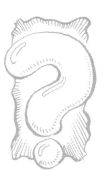

1. Yes.
    The Bach Flower Remedies are *complementary* medicines because they can work alongside any other form of therapy being used.

2. No.
    The remedies are always selected entirely according to the personality and emotional state.

3. The Bach Flower Remedies treat emotions and not the triggers that cause them, so as long as human emotions stay the same the system will contain everything needed to bring balance to troubled minds.

4. Water Violet is for those self-sufficient, calm people who like to keep themselves to themselves and at times can appear aloof and unapproachable and over-proud.

5. No, it doesn't.
    It simply means that they are people who often cut themselves off from others – but other remedies might be needed, and as with anything else you need to look below the word 'loneliness' and find the actual emotional state the person is in. Some lonely people are lonely because they are shy (Mimulus) or because they are feeling sorry for themselves and are not much fun to be with (Willow).

6. Heather people are afraid of being left alone so they chase after others and force them to become audiences as they recount their lives at great length. Water Violet people like being left alone and dislike having to explain themselves or their actions to others – they prefer to keep their privacy and keep their distance.

7. Patience.

8. Impatiens people are irritated when other people do things slowly and prevent them from getting on as quickly as they want to – in other words, irritation is rooted in impatience. Beech people are irritated by the *way* other people do things, and by mannerisms, lifestyles and so on which to them seem 'stupid' – their irritation is rooted in intolerance.

9. Cerato is for people who in their hearts know what they want, but who lack faith in their own judgement. Consequently they ask other people for their

opinions, and can end up acting against their better judgements, with predictable results.

10. No.

Water Violet is for people who tend to be like that already but find that it is causing them problems such as loneliness and isolation. You select remedies on the basis of any negative emotions you have, so you might need Agrimony if you dread being alone with your thoughts, Centaury if you lack the will-power to live your own life, and so on.

Day 5

Healing Yourself

Knowing yourself

Some people are quite happy to select remedies for their friends and family, but when it comes to choosing the ones they need themselves they quickly tie themselves up in knots. They find it harder to treat themselves than to treat others. The reason for this is simple: selecting remedies involves thinking about who you really are, and many of us are not very good at that.

For many, then, choosing the right remedies represents a journey of self-discovery. You are learning about yourself, about your reactions and feelings and fears. As you use the remedies the things you discover may surprise you.

Part of healing yourself, then, is knowing yourself. And knowledge like this is itself a healthy thing to have.

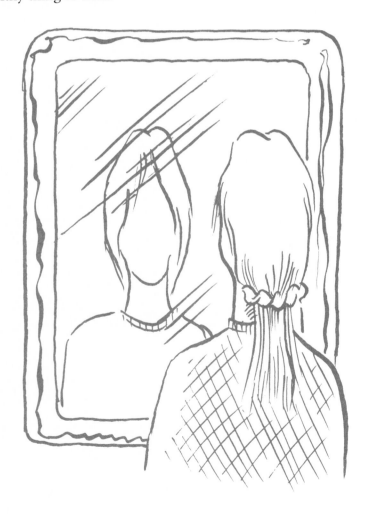

Hands-on

Maybe you have already given some
thought to what your basic type remedy is, but if you haven't you might like
to try now.

Using the list of remedy indications
in the appendix to help you, try to identify the one remedy that most closely fits the
way you normally are. You might find it useful to ask yourself the following
questions, among others:

1. Think of an occasion in the past when you have been under stress. How did
    you react?

2. Do you like lots of people around or do you prefer to be by yourself? Try
    to think of reasons for this preference.

3. What one quality that you *don't* have would you like to possess?

4. What one defect that you *do* have would you like to get rid of?

5. How do you react when other people criticise you?

6. Who do you most admire in the world, and why?

Try to narrow your choice down to one main type remedy. Some people are a
mixture of two or three, but in most cases it should be possible to isolate one
main one, even if it doesn't cover every possible facet of your personality. The
effort alone is part of the process of self-discovery.

When you have found your type remedy, write it down here.

MY TYPE REMEDY IS

Remedies for those over-sensitive to influences and ideas

WALNUT

- 'I can't get used to this new neighbourhood.'

- 'They've changed everything round at work and we don't know whether we're coming or going.'

- 'I've got an idea for a business, and I know it will work. But my uncle's company went bust last year, and he's been shaking his head over my plans. Now I'm not so sure.'

Walnut is the remedy to protect against unwanted influences and the effects of change. The aim is to help the person to cast off any external factors that may be holding him back from doing something that he wants to do. These factors might be old associations, habits or relationships, or simply the opinions of other people. And after a change has been made Walnut helps where the person feels unsettled or unhappy as a result.

Walnut is often used at significant change points in everyday life – which includes everything from teething and starting school to retirement and the menopause – to ease the transition to a new stage.

CENTAURY

- 'I'm just not very good at saying "no".'

- 'I don't go out much because I have to take care of my mother.'

- 'I always end up doing his work for him and don't have enough time left to do my own.'

The Centaury person is kind and gentle, and wants to be of service to others. Her tendency is to say 'yes' to every request. This only becomes a problem when stronger more ruthless characters enslave the Centaury, who can be worked almost to death in the service of other people and as a result spends too little time living her own life.

The remedy is not given to change the Centaury person into something else; she will always be kind and helpful; but she will have the ability to draw a line and refuse to fall into servitude.

AGRIMONY

- 'Never mind, it'll all come out in the wash.'

- 'Look on the bright side.'

- 'Eat, drink and be merry.'

The flippant remark seeking to make light of a crisis is a typical Agrimony response. Agrimony people put a cheerful mask on their inner torment. Nothing seems to disturb their good humour, but in their negative state the dark side is repressed and ignored and never integrated into the rest of life. Because of this the Agrimony suffers torment in quiet moments when there is nothing to distract him, and when the mask finally cracks he can veer dramatically into a state of utter hopelessness and distress.

The remedy is given to allow the Agrimony person to laugh at his problems but deal with them at the same time. Instead of hiding behind his good humour, he can use it to bring light to the dark times.

– CASE HISTORY –

Alan has just been talking to his girlfriend on the phone. She has told him that their relationship is over. She has been seeing someone else. Alan doesn't feel angry at her so much as numbed: he can't believe this is happening and none of it seems real. He has made up his mind to go out for a walk, but he keeps wandering round the house, forgetting what he was looking for.

- Star of Bethlehem for the shock of the bad news.

- Clematis to help him to stay anchored in the present reality and bring him back to himself.

- Both these remedies are in Rescue Remedy, which would also be a good choice.

– CASE HISTORY –

Sandy's father wants her to study for an arts degree because that's what he did when he was at university. She has always preferred science, but she is a quiet person and tends to do what others want, so when he gives her the application forms for a place reading English and Fine Art she fills them out and sends them in just to please him.

- Centaury to help Sandy to say no to her father.

HOLLY

- 'I hate her.'

- 'I can't help it, I just feel insanely jealous of her and it's eating me up.'

- 'They're up to something – I know they are.'

Holly is the remedy for very negative emotions directed towards others, such as jealousy, hatred, suspicion, spite and envy. It is often thought of as the remedy for anger, and in some cases it is – but only where the anger is the result of one of the emotions mentioned. Holly can be usefully compared with Willow, which is for resentment. It could be said that where Willow smoulders, Holly burns.

People in a Holly state are suffering from the thoughts that attack them. Holly helps to turn their thoughts into positive ones. Instead of being eaten up with hatred they can look on the world with a more generous eye, and as a result their suffering is eased.

– CASE HISTORY –

Richard has been knocked off course. 'I thought I knew what I wanted to do, and I've started to do it, but after seeing that programme on TV I'm not so sure anymore.'

- Walnut to help him resist outside influences and follow his own goals.

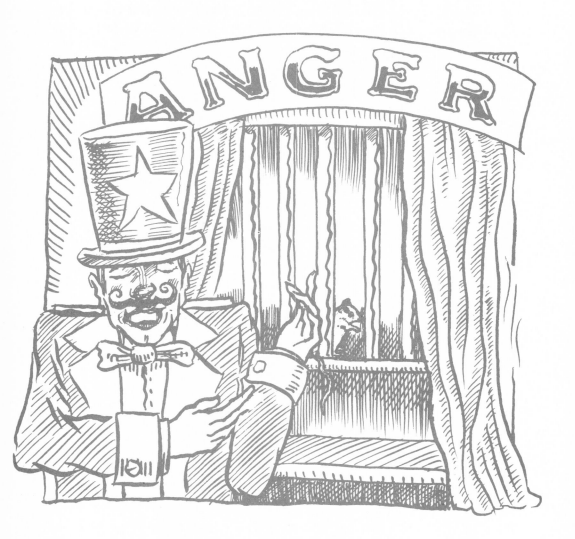

Exercise 5a

You are suffering from stress. But what are you suffering from? Look at the stressful situations and the list of remedies below, and select a single remedy for each situation. (Where you have not yet covered a remedy, brief indications have been given to help you.)

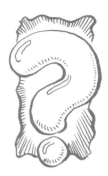

I'm under stress because …

1) … I've got a lot of responsibilities and I just took on some more. I don't know if I can cope.

2) … there have been some redundancies at work and I'm scared I may be next.

3) … people ask me to do things for them and I find it hard to say no.

4) … I'm passionately interested in this and find it hard to switch off.

5) … I can't do things as well as other people.

6   … I worry all the time.

— CASE HISTORY —

Mary's son is about to start at school for the first time. Roger is a bright, confident little boy, but Mary is convinced that he will be bullied and unhappy. As the day approaches her nervousness communicates itself to him, and instead of looking forward to his first day at school he starts to worry about it all the time. He is very anxious and isn't sleeping well.

- Red Chestnut to help Mary stop worrying unnecessarily about Roger's welfare.

- For Roger, Mimulus for his anxiety and White Chestnut for the constant worry.

- Walnut might also be useful too for both of them: to help Roger resist the influence of his mother's nervousness and to help Mary get used to the changes in her life caused by his starting school.

7) … I set myself high standards and stick to them.

8) … my ungrateful sons are neglecting me.

9) … I don't know what to do with my life.

10) … my son has got diabetes and I worry about him.

11) … I can't make up my mind about anything.

I think I'll take some …

a) … Wild Oat

b) … Scleranthus

c) … White Chestnut (for constant, repetitive, worrying thoughts)

d) … Vervain

e) … Elm (for the crisis of confidence caused by taking on too much respon-
    sibility)

f) … Chicory

g) … Mimulus

h) … Larch (for lack of confidence that prevents attempts at success)

i) … Centaury

j) … Red Chestnut

k) … Rock Water

– CASE HISTORY –

Heather has given up red meat and drinks a single glass of wine every night, whether she wants a drink or not, because it is good for her. She exercises every other day, but although she is taking part in a lot of sports she is too concerned about her performance to enjoy herself very much.

- Rock Water to help her be kinder to herself and take pleasure in pleasure.

Answers to exercise 5a

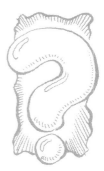

1.	e)	7.	k)
2.	g)	8.	f)
3.	i)	9.	a)
4.	d)	10.	j)
5.	h)	11.	b)
6.	c)		

Looking beyond the words

We all know that different people can use different words to describe the same thing, so that for example the same lost feeling might be described as confusion, helplessness or insecurity.

It is not so obvious, however, that the same word can be used by different people to label entirely different emotions. You might say that you can't stand your neighbour, for example: but what do you really mean? Are you frightened of him (Mimulus) or is it that you can't stand the way he behaves (Beech)? Perhaps it's his slow, deliberate manner that annoys (Impatiens) or it may be his political opinions that leave you burning with righteous indignation (Vervain). On the other hand, you may be jealous (Holly) or simply be the kind of person who likes his own company, so that your neighbour's real fault in your eyes is that he is too friendly (Water Violet).

As well as learning the keywords for the remedies, then, it's a good idea to look at how those keywords relate to the words you commonly use to describe your feelings.

— CASE HISTORY —

Vincent runs his own company and thinks of himself as a hard-headed businessman. He knows his own mind and expects others to agree with his methods. Anyone who doesn't soon finds himself out of work.

- Vine to help Vincent lead without bullying.

Exercise 5b

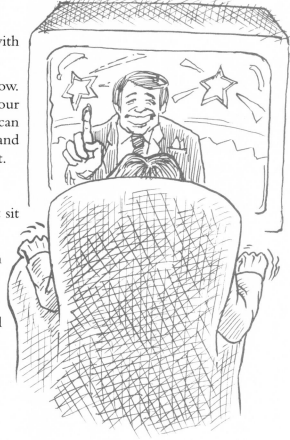

How would you describe the following two emotions? Pick the phrase you would be most likely to use and then identify a remedy for this feeling...

1. Whenever you turn on the television and see this particular comedian you feel as if someone is scratching the inside of your stomach. You have to turn off or switch over. It's something about his voice and the way he smiles that stupid smile all the time. Telling your friend about it, what would *you* say?

    a) I hate him

    b) He drives me crazy

    c) I can't stand him

    d) I've got no patience with him

2. Your driving test is tomorrow. There are butterflies in your stomach. You know you can drive but you feel uneasy and very nervous about the test.

    a) I'm terrified

    b) I'm jumpy – I just can't sit still

    c) My nerves are all on edge

    d) I feel like running away and hiding until it's all over

Answers to exercise 5b

There are no right or wrong answers to the first part of this exercise. No matter what words you would use to express the emotion the emotion itself is the same. The important thing is being able to translate the feelings described into the terminology Dr Bach used to describe the remedies. If you did this correctly you will probably have selected Beech for the first feeling and Mimulus for the second.

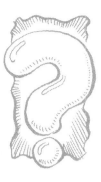

Physician, heal thyself

Edward Bach was only 50 when he died. Sometimes people ask why he wasn't able to use the flower remedies to cure himself. But in fact he did cure himself, for nearly 20 years.

Bach was turned down for military service in 1914 because of his poor state of health, but this did not stop him from working night and day at the University College Hospital. In July 1917 he suffered a severe haemorrhage and collapsed. He was suffering from cancer, and was operated on at once. When he regained consciousness after the operation he was told that the cancer would almost certainly spread and that he would be dead inside three months. But as soon as he was able to he returned to his work, and as the months went by and he found his strength returning he realised that his sense of purpose and his commitment to his work had helped him recover.

Bach believed that everyone's life had a purpose, although people often got lost on the way. By helping us recognise and feel comfortable with our true selves, the remedies can help us to rediscover our true purpose in life, which in turn brings about a return to health. This is true healing.

– CASE HISTORY –

Passed over for promotion, George responds by moaning to anyone who'll listen about the injustice of if all. Inside he actually seems quite pleased to have found something to complain about.

- Willow to help him feel more generous and positive about himself and others.

I want to make it as simple as this: 'I am hungry, I will go and pull a lettuce from the garden for my tea; I am frightened and ill, I will take a dose of Mimulus.'

QUOTED BY NORA WEEKS,
THE MEDICAL DISCOVERIES OF EDWARD BACH, PHYSICIAN

Dr Bach's discoveries were completed by August 1935; just over a year later, on 27th November 1936, he died. The cause of death was certified as heart failure. There were still traces of the cancer that should have killed him 19 years earlier. But in dying in his own time and having completed the work he was born to do, Edward Bach died a healthy man.

Hands-on

As we have seen, many people find it very difficult to look at themselves in the same objective way that they can look at others. It can help in such cases to get a second opinion.

Look again at the first project in this chapter, in which you defined your type remedy. Ask a friend who knows you well the following questions. Read them out to him or her and write down the answers you get:

1. Think of an occasion in the past when I was under stress. How did I react?

2. Do you think I like lots of people around or do I prefer to be by myself? Why do you think I am like this?

3. What one essential quality do I lack?

4. What is the worst defect in my personality?

5. How do I react when other people criticise me?

6. Who do you think I model myself on, and why?

When you have the answers to these questions try to analyse the response

> **WARNING**
>
> If you are uncomfortable with the idea of this project then don't do it. You can always come back to it when you are ready.

dispassionately, as if it has nothing to do with you. Again, try as hard as you can to narrow down the choice to one main type remedy, and when you have the answer write it down here:

MY TYPE REMEDY IS

Is the answer the same as it was in the previous project? If not, how do you account for the difference – and who has got closer to the real you?

Quick quiz

Once more the answers can be found immediately after the quiz.

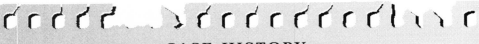

1. What are the two main indications for Walnut?

2. Why do you think Dr Bach wanted his remedies to be used as part of everyday life?

3. What is the remedy for stress?

4. What is a Centaury person like?

5. What is wrong with giving, say, 18 or 19 remedies at once?

6. What is the remedy for anger?

7. What is the *positive* quality provided by taking Mimulus?

– CASE HISTORY –

Sheila is 50. She failed her first and only driving test when she was 31, and she won't try again because she is convinced she will fail again.

- Larch to give her the confidence to try.

It is those who make an effort who get well.
THE ORIGINAL WRITINGS

8. 'She'll never admit that anything's wrong, she just laughs it off, but I know that inside she's worried sick in case any of her children start taking drugs.' What two remedies might this person need?

9. When used mixed with other remedies in a treatment bottle, does Rescue Remedy count as one remedy or five?

10. Will the Bach Flower Remedies react with drugs prescribed by a GP?

Answers to the quick quiz:

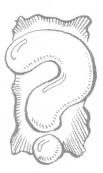

1. Walnut is for protection against outside influences, and to deal with the unsettling effects of change.

2. Because by using them as a matter of course, before any problems have a chance to take root, balance can be restored before disease itself has a chance to appear. This is using the remedies to prevent a loss of health – and in all cases prevention is better than cure.

3. There is no one remedy for stress – to select a remedy you need to look below the word and discover what it is that is putting you under stress and exactly how you are reacting to stress-producing stimuli.

4. Centaury people are over-willing to help others, and may become the slaves of more ruthless people.

5. There is nothing wrong with this if they are all needed – but in practice it is almost always possible to give a maximum of six or seven remedies, and the most Dr Bach ever gave was nine. So the chances are that in the 18 or 19 there are at least 10 that are not needed, and their presence will stop the ones that *are* needed from working so effectively.

6. Many people say Holly is the remedy for anger, but as with stress (see question 3) the real answer is that there is no one remedy for anger – it depends on what is causing the emotion. If you are angry because you are full of hatred, jealousy or spite then Holly would be the correct choice – but if yours is righteous anger you might need Vervain, impatient irritability

would need Impatiens and resentment and bitterness would indicate Willow.

7. The positive quality of Mimulus is to provide courage to allow us to face the everyday problems of life without being deflected by anxiety.

8. Agrimony for the way she is putting a cheerful face on her troubles, and Red Chestnut for her anxieties about her children.

9. It counts as a single remedy.

10. No – the only thing to be aware of is that the remedies are preserved in brandy, so medical advice should be sought before mixing them with any drugs that react strongly to alcohol. An example of this is the drug Antabuse, which is sometimes given to alcoholics in an effort to stop them from drinking.

Day 6

Healing
Others

The doctor of the future

It is possible to draw a strong analogy between the way we in the West live and the way we drive. We go too fast, taking little heed of danger signs and near misses. We take little account of the effects our passage has on other people. We assume that we are protected from the natural world, and only when reality comes crashing in do we crawl off to the garage and pay to be repaired.

Throughout the twentieth century there has been a tendency to see doctors as over-qualified garage mechanics. People limp into the surgery, suffering from the effects of years of physical and mental abuse, and expect the doctor to straighten out the knocks for them, usually so that they can go back to living their out-of-balance lives exactly as they were doing before. We break, and the doctor fixes us.

Seen from the perspective of the doctor this can be a disheartening prospect – but it also has its own subtle attractions, for in this scenario the doctor is a uniquely powerful individual. He – and it usually is a he – is given full responsibility for the health of hundreds. His power and authority are rarely questioned, and people come to him as to someone who has all the answers. The doctor doesn't just help and advise; he also *prescribes* to a *patient*.

In helping others with the Bach Flower Remedies, there are no prescribers and no patients. This is because the remedies are a self-help system, and Dr Bach's aim was reflected in the title of one of his books, *Heal Thyself*, in which he talks about the role that doctors will play in the future. The first duty of the future physician will be 'to assist the patient to a knowledge of himself'. The administering of remedies is only the second duty.

PRESCRIBING AND PATIENTS

The verb 'to prescribe' has a number of related meanings. In the weaker sense it can mean 'to advise the use of something' or 'to recommend something as being of benefit'. But it can also mean 'to impose or lay down', and whichever meaning is taken there is always a hint of authority and superiority: the person doing the prescribing assumes power over and responsibility for the person being prescribed to.

The word 'patient' also has its own rather negative connotations. A patient in a medical sense is someone who is receiving medical treatment – in other words someone in a passive role. And patients have to be patient: they have to have the ability to wait calmly and quietly to be attended to. They have to endure. But they do not have to take charge of themselves.

A FISHY STORY

What would you do if you saw a man dying of hunger next to a pool full of fish? You could catch a fish for him. Or you could teach him how to fish so that he can keep going after you have moved on.

When you help others with the remedies, then, it can be useful to think of yourself as a teacher. Don't just select remedies for people: explain what you have selected and why. Try to explain also a little about how the remedies work. Suggest ways that the people you are helping might go on to learn a little more about them and perhaps begin to apply them in their own lives. That way you are not just helping others — you are helping them to help themselves.

Remedies for despondency or despair

LARCH

- 'I wish I could do that – but I can't.'

- 'I won't be able to do it so there's no point trying.'

- 'I'm going to fail.'

People in a Larch state lack the confidence to try anything because they think they are going to fail. Having no confidence they miss opportunities. They don't do themselves justice because they are expecting things to go wrong. They fail to throw themselves whole-heartedly into life.

The positive Larch state is one of confidence, so that the person can try things and not worry over success or failure. In the words of Kipling's poem *If*, Larch people in their positive state are able to

…meet with Triumph and Disaster
And treat those two impostors just the same

ELM

- 'I just seem to be drowning in work and I'm not sure if I can cope any more.'

- So many people rely on me. Sometimes it all gets a bit much.'

Elm people don't lack confidence to try things in the way Larch people do – if anything they try to do too much, taking on more and more responsibilities until

Changes in our minds will guide us clearly to the remedy we need.
THE ORIGINAL WRITINGS

they are suddenly assailed by self-doubt. The Elm state is a crisis of confidence, then, and attacks people who are normally capable and confident.

The Elm remedy helps to resolve these temporary losses of confidence so that the Elm person can get on with her life, and know and plan for her limits.

OAK

- This hasn't worked; this hasn't worked either; now I'll try that.'

Oak people are similar to Elm types in that they are very good at coping with things; but unlike their Elm cousins they never doubt their strength or endurance. They are the tortoises in Aesop's fable who plod on step by step, never giving up until they reach their goal, relying on their enormous strength and solidity to keep them going through every adversity. The danger is that their determination can lead them to over-extend their physical strength when they get too fixed on their plodding progress. At such times the remedy is used to set them back on an even keel where they can see the need to rest now and again.

CRAB APPLE

- 'I hate the way I look.'
- 'I can't leave the house in the morning without giving it a good clean first.'
- 'I feel dirty.'

— CASE HISTORY —

Cate wants to leave her current firm and take up the offer of a better job in another town. But she has made some mistakes in her life and now doesn't trust herself to choose the right path. She asks her friends what they would do, and ends up more confused than ever.

- Cerato to help Cate trust her own decisions.

Crab Apple is the cleansing remedy. It is used to cleanse anything — mental or physical — that you don't like about yourself, including the feeling of being contaminated that can arise when you are ill. This is the aspect of this remedy that is being called on when it is included in the Rescue Cream.

People in a Crab Apple state may dislike their appearances and may also feel repugnance at normal bodily functions such as eating and excretion. By extension, compulsive orderliness, cleanliness and hand-washing are also classic Crab Apple traits, and a real Crab Apple type can be incapable of sitting in a room with a picture hung slightly askew on the wall — he will have to get up and straighten it.

PINE

- 'It's all my fault.'

- 'It was her decision, but I blame myself.'

Pine is for people who blame themselves for their own mistakes and for the mistakes of others. Often Pine people are actually very conscientious, but they are rarely satisfied with their achievements and always looking for faults in themselves.

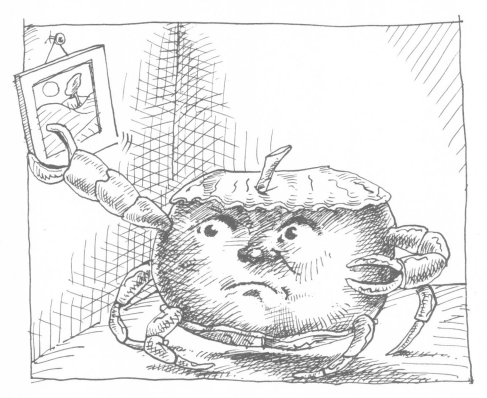

Before almost all complaints there is usually a time of not being quite fit or a bit run down: that is the time to treat our condition, get fit and stop things going further.

THE ORIGINAL WRITINGS

Even if they are right to feel guilty Pine people need to learn from their mistakes and move on. This they cannot do in the negative Pine state, so their guilt turns poisonous unless the remedy is used to help them out of the trap. Where they were not to blame in the first place the remedy helps them to see things in their proper perspective and accept and allocate responsibility in a more balanced way.

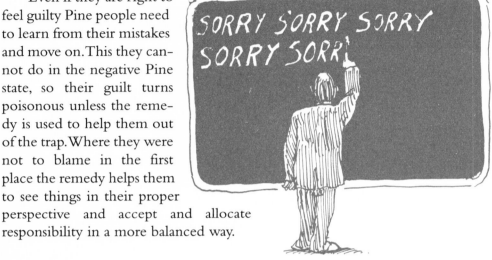

WILLOW

- 'I deserve better than this.'

- 'It's not fair.'

- 'It's all their fault.'

Pine people blame themselves for everything that goes wrong; Willow people always blame others even where they themselves are at fault. People in this state feel self-pity and resentment. They begrudge the successes and triumphs of other people and rarely have a good word to say about them.

The remedy is used to help Willow people to feel more generous towards others and more objective about their own mental state. Only when they can take some responsibility for their predicament can they start to climb out to a better life.

SWEET CHESTNUT

- 'I've tried everything and there really is no way out.'

- 'I'm trapped in total darkness.'

This is the remedy for people who have explored every alternative in their search for a way through their difficulties and now feel that they have reached the end of the road, a point where there is nowhere left to go. This is a bleak and terrible feeling, and not surprisingly the great despair often felt by those who have lost loved ones is also a Sweet Chestnut state.

Sweet Chestnut can't work miracles and make the person's problems disappear. But it will lend courage and fortitude so that hope can live again. The sufferer can find a peaceful place from which to look forward.

STAR OF BETHLEHEM

- 'I feel stunned.'

- 'This can't be happening.'

Like Sweet Chestnut, Star of Bethlehem is often associated with bereavement. It is the remedy for shock and for the great sense of loss and grief that can go along with it.

Perhaps it is because Star of Bethlehem is an important ingredient of Rescue Remedy that people sometimes think of it as a crisis remedy, for use in the here and now. But it can be used also for shocks and losses that were experienced long ago in the past and which have never been satisfactorily dealt with. In all cases the effect of this remedy is to allow the person to regain balance. Once this has been achieved, the events that knocked the personality off course can be coped with more effectively.

Exercise 6a

How would you describe the following emotion? Pick the phrase you would be most likely to use and then identify the remedy for the feeling it describes.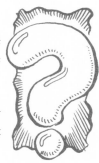

- When you stand in front of the mirror you feel you are ugly and unattractive. Because of this you feel unhappy about yourself and who you are.

  a) I hate myself

  b) I disgust myself

  c) Nobody likes me

  d) I'm useless

It is not the disease that matters: it is the patient.
THE ORIGINAL WRITINGS

Answers to exercise 6a

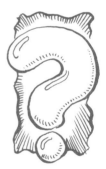

You should have selected Crab Apple for the feeling – how you described it is up to you.

Listening to others

When you are helping your friends to select remedies, you will of course listen to what they say. It goes without saying.

Well, it should do. But some of us actually find it very difficult to go for any length of time without saying something. We impose our ideas and interpretations, we hedge and direct the responses we hear and the result is that we don't actually find out the things we really need to know.

Exercise 6b

In the following short dialogue Ann is trying to help Victor, who is having trouble sleeping. See if you can spot five separate problems with the way Ann approaches this conversation, then turn the page to see some improvements in place.

ANN: What do you think about when you can't sleep? Do you have trouble relaxing generally?

– CASE HISTORY –

Ian is driving too fast with an empty petrol tank because he is late for a meeting. In his rush to get there he has decided to take a chance on there being enough petrol. He loses. The engine dies and he sits furious in his car, cursing the delay.

- Impatiens to help him see the sense in planning and not always being in a rush.

— CASE HISTORY —

After ten hours' sleep Cathy gets into work and sits at her desk and looks at her in-tray, and she could weep for tiredness.

- Hornbeam to help her overcome her exhaustion at the thought of the work she has to do.

VICTOR: Well, I don't get to relax much, so …

ANN: When is it that you have trouble relaxing – at work or after work, say, at the end of the day?

VICTOR: It's during the day, mostly.

ANN: Do you like your job?

VICTOR: Well, yes, I suppose so …

ANN: Is it a responsible job?

VICTOR: Quite responsible, yes.

ANN: I'd say you're a reliable sort but you've maybe taken on a bit too much recently and it's knocked your confidence. Try some Elm and let's see if that helps.

— CASE HISTORY —

Gwen's husband has left her. She is convinced that it's her own fault because she has got so fat and out of shape – although unaccountably she is still a size 10, just as she has always been.

- Crab Apple for her dislike of her own appearance.

Answers to exercise 6b

Here are the five things wrong with Ann's approach:

1. She starts out by asking two separate questions in quick succession, leaving no space for an answer to the first and immediately putting Victor under pressure.

2. She interrupts Victor when he pauses in his first reply, not allowing him to expand on what he has said.

3. She asks a 'double question'; in other words she expects Victor to select between two possible replies and doesn't let him give his own answer.

4. She asks a closed question, to which Victor can only answer yes or no.

5. She sums up and selects Elm far too quickly: there is no evidence whatsoever that Elm is needed, it is just an assumption she has made.

So how could Ann have approached this? She could have:

• Asked open questions – questions that cannot be answered with a 'yes' or 'no', so that Victor would have had a chance to express himself.

• Allowed Victor time to think, pause and answer, and not filled in all the silences herself.

• Asked one question at a time.

– CASE HISTORY –

Karen is a dedicated and very capable health visitor working in a tough inner-city area. She is responsible for over 200 families, many of them living below the poverty line. When one of 'her' children is taken into care she suddenly feels as if she has failed, and for the first time she is depressed by the burden of responsibility on her. She's not sure she can cope any more.

• Elm for the temporary loss of confidence.

- Asked more questions to give Victor a chance to confirm or reject the remedies she was considering.

Most important of all, she should have:

- Listened more and talked less.

Let's see how the conversation might have gone if Ann had taken this advice on board:

ANN: What do you think about when you can't sleep?

VICTOR: It's mainly about work. I got passed over for promotion, which is typical really. That sort of thing always happens to me. Other people seem to do all right even though they do half the work I do. I'm not a complainer but it does get me down.

ANN: How are you about relaxing generally?

VICTOR: Not very good. It's just one of those things that I'm not very good at.

ANN: When is it that you mostly have trouble relaxing?

VICTOR: Weekdays. The weekends aren't so bad, but ... it's in the week, in the

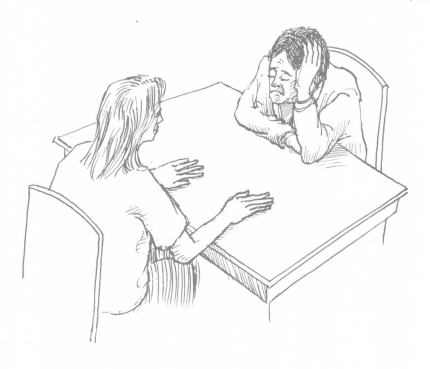

The illness of yesterday is of yesterday, and of no interest or importance now. What we have to treat is the present state of the patient.

THE ORIGINAL WRITINGS

early morning, when I know I have to get up and go back to the same job. Just thinking about it knocks all the fight out of me.

ANN: When you say it knocks all the fight out of you, how do you feel exactly?

VICTOR: You know, tired, jaded, like I'd rather stay lying around in bed than have to face the day.

ANN: Is there anything you like about your job?

VICTOR: The job's all right as far as it goes. I suppose it's the people at work more than anything. I can't respect them. My boss, for example – she hasn't had half the education I have yet there she is in charge of the department.

ANN: If you could do another job, anything you wanted, what would you choose?

VICTOR: I don't know. I think I'm a bit old to change track now. I always want-ed to be a toy-maker, you know, work with wood, but anything like that would be bound to fail with the way things are now, so many busi-nesses going bust and so on.

ANN: Have you thought about starting off in your spare time?

VICTOR: I'm just one of those people who can't do things like that. It'd all go belly-up and I'd end up out of pocket, so why bother?

ANN: I think there are three remedies that would be helpful to you …

FURTHER EXERCISE

What remedies do you think Ann has chosen? See the end of this chapter for my suggestions!

While you're thinking about this, think also about how Ann should explain to Victor what each remedy is for. Is there a right and a wrong way to tell peo-ple why you are giving them a particular remedy?

Exercise 6c

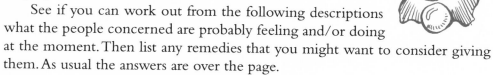

As well as listening to people, a lot of information can be gained by looking at how people act, how they sit or stand, the gestures they use and their appearance. These are not fail-safe indicators, but they can certainly suggest an initial line of enquiry.

See if you can work out from the following descriptions what the people concerned are probably feeling and/or doing at the moment. Then list any remedies that you might want to consider giving them. As usual the answers are over the page.

1. Adam is almost lying on his chair, with his hands behind his head and his legs stretched out in front of him. His face is half-turned to the ceiling, but he glances down at you a great deal, sometimes staring.

2. Beatrice sits very erect and rigid in her seat, with her fists clenched and her arms folded tightly across her chest and her feet and knees pressed tightly together.

3. Claire is leaning towards you while you talk, and nods her head when you make a point. Her legs are crossed so that the top leg points towards you.

4. Derek's head is thrust forward and he is looking directly into your eyes without blinking. He is white-faced and his hands are at his side and clenched.

5. Edward is standing up, but his shoulders are rounded and his neck and head droop towards the floor. He speaks in a monotone.

— CASE HISTORY —

Vera has been suffering from headaches, and they've been getting worse. She won't go to see a doctor because she says it runs in her family: her father and his father both had the same thing, and just as nobody could help them, so nothing can be done for her.

- Gorse to overcome her hopelessness so that she can see a path out of her difficulties and follow it.

A WORD OF WARNING

Body language can be misleading. For example, imagine someone frowning all through your conversation. He could be unsure of what you are saying. He could be concentrating hard so as not to miss anything. Or he could have a headache. The only way to know which is correct, is to ask.

Answers to exercise 6c

1. Adam probably feels rather superior to you, and doesn't appear to be very interested in you or what you are saying. It isn't possible to suggest any remedies at the moment, although you might put a question mark against Vine.

2. Beatrice is very tense, and ready to defend herself against any approach on your part. Rock Water could be indicated, or Mimulus or Beech or Vervain or many others, but of course more information is needed.

3. Claire is interested by what you are saying and is encouraging you to continue. From her body language alone, she seems well balanced and not in need of any remedies.

4. Derek is very aggressive and may be on the point of using violence. Cherry Plum would help him to keep control of himself, and Holly might be appropriate if hatred was the cause of his aggression, although other remedies like Vine, Beech and even Impatiens also need to be considered.

5. Edward is probably depressed and despondent – although he could equally well be exhausted. Hornbeam, Willow, Elm, Sweet Chestnut, Gorse and Gentian are probably among the first to consider. (If you looked in the Appendix you might also have thought about Olive, which will be covered in the next chapter.)

How long do the remedies take to work?

People often ask how long it will take for the remedies to work. The answer is 'it depends'...

They work very quickly when it comes to acute situations that are not rooted in long-standing imbalances. So for example if you are feeling tired after a hard day's work and you take some Olive, you should feel the benefits very quickly. And Rescue Remedy, which is especially formulated for emergency use, often has very dramatic results.

Where the problem being addressed has been going on for some time or there are fundamental imbalances involved it may take some time to get to the root of them. Everyone is different, so it is hard to generalise, but a useful rule of thumb is that you should have noticed some improvement after about three weeks. This is about the time that a treatment bottle will last if used regularly, so the end of a treatment bottle provides a natural opportunity to review the selection of remedies to see if other remedies are now needed as well as or instead of the ones originally selected. But with very deep-rooted problems it can take even longer to see definite changes, so if you review a selection and still feel the same remedies are needed, don't be afraid to go on giving them.

WHO NOTICES THE CHANGE?

Sometimes when you are taking remedies you are the last person to notice that they are working. Instead loved ones, friends, or colleagues at work will remark quite innocently how much happier, calmer, or whatever you are, and wonder what tremendous event in your life can have caused such a change.

There are a very few people who at some level seem not to want to get better. They may have found a way of coping that leaves them out of balance but at least allows them to get through their lives. Remember that in the end every person is responsible for his or her own life: you can offer help to people, but if it is refused you shouldn't and can't force them to take it.

Finally, people sometimes ask when it is safe to stop taking the remedies. The answer is that it is *safe* to stop taking them at any time, since they are not habit-forming and do not cause dependence. And there is no need to go on taking them in case the problem comes back: as soon as the problems you are addressing are no longer there, you can stop the treatment. In practice people find that they quite naturally forget to take the drops when they no longer need them.

Peeling the onion

As we go through our lives, things happen to us which can knock us off course. Emotional problems build up over time, layer by layer, until the original emotional cause can be quite hidden.

It can be uncomfortable or even dangerous to try to cut straight to the hidden heart of things, particularly where people are not ready to face issues that might lie buried deep in their minds. The remedies are gentler because they approach the problem layer by layer, starting from the outside. By the time the centre is reached the person taking them is ready to face it and deal with it calmly.

This is why when selecting the remedies you should always choose them entirely on the basis of what you see. There is no need for in-depth analysis or occult or psychologically invasive techniques.

If you treat only what you see you will find that the remedies you choose will be able to work without being muddied by other unnecessary remedies. And as the remedies do their work hidden negative states will become clearer by themselves. Be lazy, then – let the remedies do the work.

TREATING WHAT YOU SEE

When you select remedies for someone all kinds of remedies can pop into mind. Colin says he's feeling sorry for himself (Willow) – maybe that also means he is feeling guilty about something (Pine) and full of regrets about the past (Honeysuckle)?

This might be true, and if you were talking to Colin you could ask him questions that would help you decide whether or not Pine and Honeysuckle would indeed be useful remedies. But if you only have a limited amount of information that is what you need to use as a basis for selection – and not your guesses or memories of the way you felt when a similar thing happened to you.

Hands-on

Now to try out your skills on someone else! For this project, pick someone who you know reasonably well but who is not a very close friend – a distant relative might be a good choice, or a casual acquaintance or a work colleague. Then proceed as follows: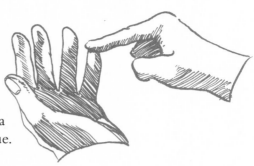

PART ONE:

Explain to your partner that you are going to try to select some Bach Flower Remedies for him/her. Find a quiet half-hour when you will not be disturbed and conduct a simple consultation.

Try to remember the following points during the interview:

- Your partner might never have heard of the Bach Flower Remedies before, so in the first few minutes explain what they are and underline the fact that they are safe.

- You should listen more than you talk.

- Make sure that your partner can *see* that you are listening.

- Try to ask open questions that encourage your partner to enlarge on the answer.

- Look for clues about your partner's feelings from his or her gestures, posture, appearance and tone of voice.

- When you think of a remedy that might be helpful, ask questions to check if it is the right one.

You can refer to the list of remedies in the Appendix at the back of this book if you need to, but try not to do this too much as it might get in the way of your conversation. For the same reason, don't make too many notes, although you might find it helpful to jot down ideas for remedies and further questions as you go.

At the end of the half hour, make up a treatment bottle containing the remedies you selected and arrange a follow-up interview in about three weeks' time. Remember to explain why you have selected those particular remedies.

I consider it the duty and privilege of any physician to teach the sick and others how to heal themselves.

THE ORIGINAL WRITINGS

PART TWO:

In about three weeks, meet your partner again and check that the remedies have been taken regularly. Ask your partner if he or she feels better or worse.

Continue as before to discuss your partner's mental state as it is at the moment, in particular noting:

- Have there been any material changes in his or her circumstances since the last interview?

PRACTITIONER TRAINING

The material in this chapter is designed to help you to select remedies for your friends and family.

If you want to practise with the Bach Flower Remedies professionally, see the section 'Where to Go from Here', at the end of this book.

- What emotional changes have there been since last time?

- Are any of the remedies you chose last time no longer needed?

- Is there now a need for any new remedies?

During the conversation, make an effort to teach a little about the remedies as you go. Again, make up a new treatment bottle and explain any changes in the selection made.

– CASE HISTORY –

June hates her job. Every lunch time she wanders into the park to get away from the office and sits on a bench lost in daydreams of fame and fortune. She doesn't do anything to make her dreams come true.

- Clematis to bring her back to the present so she can take action instead of just dreaming.

PART THREE:

Now the second interview is over, think about the following, if possible with the help of your partner in the consultation:

- Which interview was easier for you: the first or the second? Why?

- Which interview was easier for the other person? Again, why?

- Look back over this chapter at the various hints on selecting remedies for other people. Is there anything you didn't do that might have helped? Is there anything you did that you would not do next time?

Exercise 6d

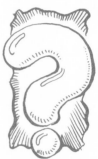

When you are explaining to someone why they should take the remedies you have selected it is important to do so in a tactful way. In your own words, explain to the following people why you are giving them the remedies listed. Then compare your explanations with those suggested afterwards.

1. Your neighbour has talked about himself and his parking ticket for over two hours. You've just been declared bankrupt but you've barely got a word in. Tell him why you are giving him some Heather.

2. Your mother comes round every other evening and insists on cooking dinner for you and your husband. Explain why you think she needs some Chicory.

3. Your colleague at work blames everyone but himself for his many errors. He is full of self-pity and compares his own ill fortune with the undeserved luck of other people. See if you can persuade him to take some Willow.

4. Your friend's husband is insanely jealous of her and hardly lets her out of his sight. He is an aggressive man and has said on a couple of occasions that he hates his wife's friends — including, presumably, you. How would you take advantage of one of his better days to get him to try some Holly?

5. His wife, your friend, has got to the point where she hardly seems to have a will of her own any more. You have heard her described as a doormat, and in truth she usually does what other people want her to do. What kinder way can you find to describe the situation and explain the benefits of taking Centaury?

KEEPING MUM

You might think that it is easier not to bother explaining. The problems start when someone decides to look up the indications afterwards and is less than pleased to find that Beech, Willow and Heather mean that you think him an intolerant, self-pitying bore!

To avoid this happening it's probably best to explain remedy indications right from the start. Doing this also helps people to learn a little about how to choose remedies, so that they will be better able to select for themselves.

Answers to exercise 6d

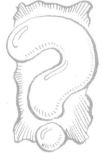

The general rule is to stress the positive side of the remedies (i.e. the aim of taking the remedies, rather than the problem that causes you to take them in the first place). You might also refer back to things said during the conversation – so if your neighbour has said himself that he knows that he talks too much, then it is OK for you to remind him of that when you are describing what Heather is for. But these are guidelines rather than hard and fast rules. It's quite possible that your answers will improve on these suggestions:

1. I'm giving you some Heather to help you to get your problems into perspective. That way they won't seem so overwhelming and you'll be able to enjoy the company of others more.

– CASE HISTORY –

Jill is 18 and has just left home for the first time to go to university. She is having trouble adjusting to life in a shared house with other students, and feels very down and homesick.

*   Walnut to help her to adjust to the change in her life.

*   Honeysuckle to turn her mind away from the past so she can enjoy the present more.

2. I know it must be hard now that the children have flown the coop. I think the Chicory will help you see that your family hasn't gone, it's just spreading and growing.

3. You've maybe been a bit down in the mouth recently, but that's perfectly normal. The Willow is just to help you to feel more positive about life — and I think you'll find the people at work will appreciate you more because of it.

4. Deep down I think you are a generous person, but that side of you can be hidden sometimes when you feel the world is against you. The Holly will help you to show your wife how much you love her in a more effective way.

5. You're someone who likes to help others, and there's nothing wrong with that. But if people are beginning to take you for granted and trying to push you around, Centaury will help you to draw the line and keep some time and space for yourself.

Mount Vernon

Early in 1934 Dr Bach left Cromer, in Norfolk, where he had spent the winter. He was looking for a village house, somewhere quiet, where he would be able to complete his research and where his work could find its spiritual and material home. After looking around he decided in April 1934 on the village of Sotwell, where he rented a modest two-storey cottage called Mount Vernon.

All the last 19 of the 38 flower remedies were found in the lanes and countryside around Mount Vernon — and to his delight Bach discovered that almost all of the first 19 were also to be found locally. Bach dug and scattered seed over the garden at Mount Vernon, and furnished the house with tables, chairs and bookcases of his own design — there wasn't enough money to buy furniture new.

Dr Bach died in November 1936 and was buried in the local churchyard, a short walk from the house and garden he loved. He left his work in the hands of Nora Weeks and Victor Bullen, asking them to protect its simplicity and purity and to make it available to all of humanity — a request which they were honoured to fulfil.

In the late 1950's, having come through the difficult war years and with the Bach Flower Remedies now becoming better known, Nora and Victor were

Never let anyone give up hope of getting well.

THE ORIGINAL WRITINGS

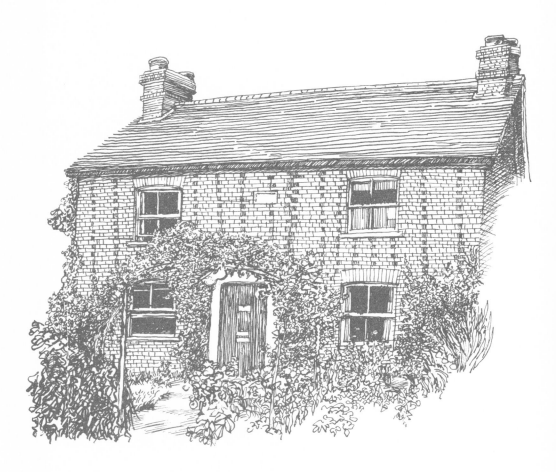

able to raise enough money through donations to buy Mount Vernon and transfer it to a trust which they had set up for the purpose. In this way they secured the house for all time to be the continuing centre of Dr Bach's work, as he had wanted.

Quick quiz

Once more the answers can be found immediately after the quiz.

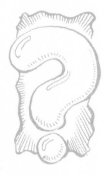

1. Larch and Elm can both be described as being 'for lack of confidence' — but what is the difference between them?

2. What are the indications for Pine?

3. If you look at yourself in the mirror and don't like your appearance, which remedy would you take?

4. What if you were suffering today because of a shock that you had ten years ago? Could you still take Star of Bethlehem?

5. When should you stop taking the remedies?

6. When is the Oak remedy needed?

7. If the Bach Flower Remedies are meant for self-help, why does the Bach Centre train professional practitioners?

8. What does 'peeling the onion' mean?

9. If you were giving your husband Wild Rose because he was apathetic, would you tell him so?

10. What is the relevance of Mount Vernon to the Bach Flower Remedies?

Answers to the quick quiz:

1. Larch is for people who lack confidence to try things, as they are convinced they are not as clever or skilful as others are and so imagine they will fail. Theirs is a fear of failure, then, which comes before they do anything. Elm people are actually confident and competent and often hold responsible positions. Theirs is a *crisis* of confidence rather than a *lack* of confidence. Typically it is caused by their taking on more than they can comfortably deal with.

2. Pine is for people who feel guilty: they blame themselves when things go wrong, whether or not the fault is really theirs.

3. Crab Apple is the remedy for people who feel there is something unclean

about them, and this can include a dislike of their own appearance.

4. Yes – although it is often used in immediate emergencies, Star of Bethlehem is just as useful for shocks in the past.

5. Quite simply, when the feelings you are treating have passed.

6. The Oak state is in most ways a positive one, and the remedy is needed only when things go too far and the determined Oak threatens to push past the natural limits of strength and on into exhaustion and collapse.

7. There are many people who are reluctant to start to heal themselves without guidance, and even people who have been using the remedies for years can encounter selection problems that respond better to the dispassionate eye of another person. A properly trained practitioner can help in both cases, especially one taught that the practitioner's job is to educate and not to prescribe.

8. It describes the process whereby treating the apparent emotional state of a person can sometimes reveal hidden layers of emotional upset underneath, which in turn have to be treated before balance can be restored.

9. It would be kinder – and he would be more likely to listen – if you told him that you were giving him Wild Rose to help him take charge of his life. Telling him he is apathetic is not likely to help matters, however true it might be!

10. Mount Vernon is the cottage where Dr Bach decided to centre his work, and the place from where the remedies have spread all over the world. The mother tinctures for the Bach Flower Remedies are still made there to this day.

Answer to extra question for exercise 6a: the remedies that Ann chose for Victor were Willow, Larch and Hornbeam.

Day 7

PUTTING IT ALL TOGETHER

Four advantages

In September 1936 Dr Bach gave a lecture in the Masonic Hall in Wallingford, a few miles away from Mount Vernon. In his introduction he outlined the particular qualities of his discoveries. This is what he said:

> The system being spoken of this evening has great advantages over others.
>
> Firstly. All the remedies are made from beautiful flowers, plants and trees of Nature: none of them are poisonous nor can do any harm, no matter how much was taken.
>
> Secondly. They are only 38 in number, which means that it is easier to find the right herb to give, than when there are very many.
>
> Thirdly. The method of choosing which remedies to give is simple enough for most people to understand.
>
> Fourthly. The cures which have been obtained have been so wonderful, that they have passed all expectations of even those who use this method...

(See *The Original Writings of Edward Bach*, edited by Judy Howard and John Ramsell.)

ONLY 38?

Although there are only 38 remedies, between them they cover every possible negative mental state. This can seem hard to understand – people are complicated things, after all, and there must be more than 38 possible states of mind.

Look at it this way: the largest number of different remedies Dr Bach ever gave at once was nine. Using this as the limit there are already well over 292,000,000 different combinations available.

Then go further: consider the fact that two people needing the same set of remedies will be experiencing the component emotions of their mental states to different degrees. In other words, if I need Willow and Beech and you do too, there might be more Willow than Beech in my mental state and more Beech than Willow in yours. So in fact the 38 remedies cover an infinite number of different mental states.

There is empirical evidence for this claim: in over sixty years no-one has ever been turned away from the Bach Centre with the words 'Sorry, Dr Bach didn't think of something for *that*!'

Once we have been given a jewel of such magnitude, nothing can deviate us from our path of love and duty to displaying its lustre, pure and unadorned to the people of the world.

THE ORIGINAL WRITINGS

Remedies for insufficient interest in present circumstances

HONEYSUCKLE

- 'All my joy lies in the past.'

- 'I remember the time when …'

Honeysuckle is for people who live in the past instead of the present. They spend much of their energy thinking about and reliving past glories – or tragedies – and because of this they do not get much out of the lives they live now.

The remedy is used to help bring people in this state back to the here and now so that they can start to live again. The positive side to Honeysuckle is being able to remember past happiness and make it part of the happiness felt in the present. Instead of feeling that all joy is past, the person can see the potential for joy in every new day.

CLEMATIS

- 'I'm sorry, I was miles away.'

- 'What did you say?'

- 'I get so wrapped up with planning what I'm going to do that I never seem to get around to doing it.'

In some ways Clematis is the opposite of Honeysuckle, for while in both cases insufficient interest is paid to the present, the Clematis person lives more in the future than in the past. Clematis people are great dreamers who tend to use up their energies in fantasy and not in the real world. On a more mundane level anyone who begins to drift into daydreams instead of concentrating on what is happening is in a Clematis state.

The remedy helps to bring the person back to the present. The great dreams of the Clematis person may then come true.

WHITE CHESTNUT

- 'I can't stop thinking about it.'

- 'It's like a record playing in my head.'

- 'I worry all the time.'

White Chestnut people don't pay attention to what they are doing either, but in their case they are prevented from doing so by worrying, insistent thoughts that seem to go round and round in their minds with no respite. The worries them- selves may be over things that may or may not happen, or they may involve replaying over and over again some scene or argument experienced during the day.

   The remedy helps to calm the worry and put the sufferer back in control of his own mind. This allows him to get on with his life in a rational way.

WILD ROSE

- 'I don't care.'

- 'That's the way it goes.'

- 'I don't mind either way.'

Wild Rose people seem apathetic and lethargic and make little or no effort to improve or learn from their lives. But they are not normally unhappy about this state of affairs – which sets them apart from people in a Hornbeam state, for example. Instead they are resigned to what happens to them and quite content to let things go and just drift.

– CASE HISTORY –

Every morning Kevin is late for work. The alarm clock goes off on time, but he always thinks 'just another five minutes...' and the next thing he knows he has overslept again. Every night he vows it won't happen again, and every morning it does.

- Chestnut Bud to help him learn from experience and stop making the same mistakes.

The remedy is used with people in this state to help them take a more active interest in the world. They will still be the same easy-going, relaxed people they always were, but they will be more interested in themselves and others, and because of this their lives will be more fulfilled.

CHESTNUT BUD

- 'I'm always getting into the same situations.'

- 'It always ends the same way.'

People in a Chestnut Bud state seem unable to make out the patterns in their own lives and in the lives of others. Instead of making a mistake and learning from it they make the same mistakes over and over again. And they can watch other people falling into an error and then, when it is their turn to act, make the same mistake themselves.

So this is the remedy for people who seem unable to learn from experience. The aim of taking it is to spare them unnecessary suffering by allowing them to profit more from events in their lives. That way they can learn and move on to a higher more competent level of life.

OLIVE

- 'It's been a hard day, and I'm exhausted.'

- 'This illness has really taken it out of me.'

Olive is for physical and mental exhaustion that has a definite cause, such as illness or working or studying too hard, or undergoing a great deal of suffering. As such it can be contrasted with Hornbeam: Olive is for tiredness after doing something, Hornbeam is for tiredness at the *thought* of doing something.

HELPERS

White Chestnut and Olive are two of the most-selected remedies in Dr Bach's system. This is because they treat symptoms that come very frequently as a result of other more basic problems.

For example, a Vervain person who has become committed to a cause may overwork to the point of exhaustion and find it very difficult to switch off and stop thinking about the same thing over and over again. Vervain is the main remedy needed, but by giving White Chestnut for the constant repetitious thoughts and Olive for the tiredness you will clear up these aspects of the problem all the sooner.

MUSTARD

- 'I feel depressed but I don't know why.'

- 'I can't see the point of anything.'

Mustard is for the kind of gloomy depression that comes out of a clear blue sky. People in this state often list all the good things there are in their life and are at a complete loss to account for their unhappiness.

The remedy is used to lift the black clouds so that people in this state can gain real joy from the good things in their lives.

Exercise 7a

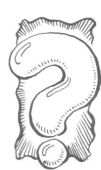

Here are brief descriptions of seven women at a particular moment in their lives. See if you can match each mental state to one of the seven remedies listed below.

THE PEOPLE:

1. Her boss is trying to tell Eve that the company is going to have to let her go, but Eve looks as if she's hardly listening. She's miles away.

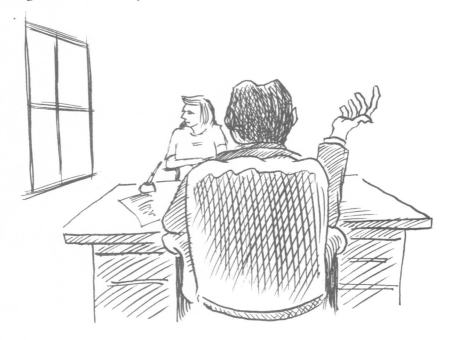

2. Eve has just been told that she is being fired, but she never liked the job much anyway, so she shrugs and goes back to her desk to finish her sandwich.

3. After losing her job, Eve went out drinking and dancing until 5 am. Now it's the morning and she's supposed to be seeing someone about a job, but she can hardly keep her eyes open.

4. While her boss is telling her the bad news, all Eve can think about is the day she started the job and how happy she was. She's sure that she'll never again feel as confident and full of future as she did then.

5. Eve's been fired before. It always comes as a surprise, although when she thinks about it her bosses always mention time keeping as a factor.

6. Eve's career is going well, she has just met a new man and her new company car arrives in the car pool tomorrow. She can't for the life of her figure out why, but she is completely down in the dumps.

7. Eve was fired at 10.30 in the morning, and by 11.30 was at home. Ever since then she's been replaying the scene in her head, thinking of all the things she should have said to her boss. She can't stop her mind re-running the whole thing, although heaven knows she's got plenty of other things to sort out.

THE REMEDIES:

A. Clematis

B. Honeysuckle

C. Wild Rose

D. Olive

E. White Chestnut

F. Mustard

G. Chestnut Bud

Our work is steadfastly to adhere to the simplicity and purity of this method of healing.

THE ORIGINAL WRITINGS

Answers to exercise 7a

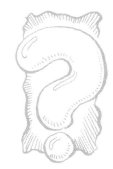

1. A.

2. C.

3. D.

4. B.

5. G.

6. F.

7. E.

The importance of simplicity

Dr Bach left his work complete, and made it as simple as possible for people to use. That's why at the end of his life he didn't concern himself with putting together ten-volume sets of his life's work, but instead condensed all he had achieved into the 32 pages of *The Twelve Healers*.

Its simplicity makes this a system of medicine that we can all use to heal our emotions. Used properly there is no need for experts or special, arcane selection techniques. And the fact that the system is complete – the fact that it covers all negative mental states – means there is no need to add thousands of new essences to the original 38.

– CASE HISTORY –

Two-year-old Jonathan is in the middle of a temper tantrum, and can't even remember why he is angry.

- Cherry Plum to help him get control of himself again.

Distortion is a far greater weapon than attempted destruction.

THE ORIGINAL WRITINGS

Exercise 7b

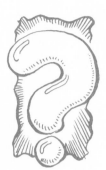

1. Which remedies do you think these two people need at the moment?

    Mr A: 'When I look back I wish I'd spent more time with my parents. I remember the Sunday dinners my mother used to cook and how she was always so pleased when I went to eat there. I don't suppose I'll ever eat as well as that again. I don't know, nothing seems as bright as it did in those days.'

    Mr B: 'Sorry, what did you say? I was daydreaming.'

2. What would you give this lady?
    'I'm an accountant. Every year about this time I have to do year-end figures for my company and every year it's the same: I just can't turn off when I get home. All the time I'm eating, watching television or trying to get to sleep I'm adding numbers up, almost as if I'm double-checking what I've been doing at work. Of course, it takes ages to get to sleep and then I'm exhausted the next day. By the time I've finished the accounts I'm ready to drop. It's my own fault, of course, because I always delay starting work until the last possible moment. I never seem to learn.'

3. Finally, what would you suggest for this person?

    'Most of the time I'm a pretty easy-going sort of guy. I like to take life as it comes, and if things don't go well it doesn't bother me really. The stupid thing is I've been really depressed this last couple of weeks when in fact there's no reason to be, or at least no reason that I can see. But that's life I suppose.'

Answers to exercise 7b

1.   Mr A needs Honeysuckle because he is reliving past plea-
     sures and regrets and not enjoying the present for itself. Mr
     B has drifted off into a world of his own and could do with
     some Clematis to bring his attention back.

2.   This lady could certainly use some White Chestnut for the
     repetitive thoughts that are troubling her and some Olive
     for her tiredness. The main remedy she needs, though, is
     Chestnut Bud. This will help her learn from her repeated crises and leave a
     little more time for the accounts next year.

3.   Wild Rose is the type remedy for this person, and Mustard will help to
     shake him out of his current motiveless depression.

Treating animals and plants

They are less likely to be defensive and they don't attempt to hide their feelings:
animals respond very well to the Bach Flower Remedies. Good reports have also
been received about treating plants.

   In both cases the main remedy used is unquestionably Rescue Remedy. This
is partly because of the difficulty involved in trying to understand what an animal is really feeling – let alone a plant. But there is also a good psychological rea-

DOSAGE FOR ANIMALS

- For small to medium sized animals, put 2 drops of individual remedies (4 of
  Rescue Remedy) into the drinking water every time it is replenished.
- Alternatively make up a treatment bottle and squirt drops from this directly
  into the animal's mouth. This is especially useful if the animal does not drink
  often enough to get the minimum dose from a water bowl.
- For larger animals, such as cows and horses, add approximately double the
  normal dosage – 8 to 10 drops of Rescue Remedy (4-5 of single remedies) to
  every bucket of water.

Incidentally, if you have two dogs which share a water bowl but you need to give
remedies to only one of them, you can still put the remedies in the bowl. If the
other dog doesn't need the same mix as the first they will simply have no effect
on it.

DOSAGE FOR PLANTS

There are a couple of ways to administer the remedies to plants.
- Add 2 drops of each individual remedy (4 of Rescue Remedy) to a spray, and spray on the plant.
- Add the same amount to the watering can and water over and around the base of the plant.

In addition, John Ramsell mentions (in *Questions and Answers*) applying Rescue Remedy Cream to the damaged trunk of a sapling — so this is another idea to bear in mind.

son, since animals and plants can be expected to react with their own versions of panic, terror, shock and loss of control to accidents and traumatic events of all kinds. These are precisely the emotions that the Rescue Remedy is formulated to deal with.

Other remedies that are commonly used with animals include Mimulus (for timidity and for specific fears), Walnut (to help them get used to new surroundings, such as a new home), Crab Apple (often dabbed onto wounds for its cleansing properties, or given in cases of parasite infestation), and Chicory (for pets who dislike not being the centre of attention all the time). Finally, cats as a whole are often spoken of as being Water Violets, and of course many are — but they can be other types as well.

Plants can benefit from Walnut and Star of Bethlehem when being replanted or repotted, while a little diluted Crab Apple can be sprayed on to help any that have been attacked by parasites. Some plants can get very sorry for themselves or seem to give up when the conditions are not right for them, and some gardeners have found Willow or Gorse to be a help at such times.

Exercise 7c

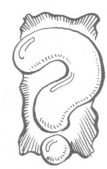

Try to think of some suitable remedies for the following animals:

1. Charlie is quite a highly strung, nervous poodle. Usually he leads a quiet life with his elderly owner, but while she is on holiday he has been packed off to a family of loud, boisterous relatives. He's having trouble adjusting.

2. Cleo isn't a kitten any more, but she still demands a great deal

of attention from her family and if she doesn't get it she is liable to rip up the curtains or scratch the furniture – she'd rather be yelled at than be ignored.

3. Bruce is supposed to be a guard dog, but any burglar would be very unlucky to catch him awake. He seems to sleep 20 hours out of 24 and when he is up he barely pays attention to what's going on around him. He seems quite happy just to eat and sleep.

4. Harry is a donkey who has been taken into a sanctuary. He is scared of people and won't let anyone get near him, but judging by the scars on his back he must have suffered a terrible beating at some time.

Answers to exercise 7c

1. Charlie could benefit from Rescue Remedy, of course, plus Mimulus for his nervous temperament and Walnut to help him adjust to the change.

2. Cleo sounds like a Chicory cat.

3. Bruce is a mix of Clematis (his sleepiness, lack of attention to the present) and Wild Rose (his acceptance of things as they are and lack of get-up-and-go).

4. Harry probably needs Mimulus and Star of Bethlehem above all, but Rescue Remedy would also be helpful.

– CASE HISTORY –

Ursula shuts herself in her bedroom and refuses to come out. She says she feels depressed, but can't give any good reason for feeling like that. Any objective observer would say that she was enjoying an especially good life.

• Mustard to help her shake off the gloom and despondency that have descended out of a clear sky.

Revision exercise 1

Fill in the blanks in the following one-sentence remedy descriptions.

1. If you keep making the same mistakes you might need _____.

2. Rock Water people are very strict with _____.

3. Someone who always laughs off problems instead of facing them needs _____.

4. The worst kind of ultimate despair and unbearable anguish calls for _____.

5. People who get depressed when things go a bit wrong need _____.

6. Rock Rose is the remedy for sheer _____.

7. When you know what you want to do but don't trust your own decision you need _____.

8. People in a _____state suffer from very negative feelings towards others, like envy, hatred, suspicion and revengeful thoughts.

9. _____ people criticise others and find it difficult to be tolerant of other ways of life.

10. If you are living in the past you need _____.

— CASE HISTORY —

Tracy is a supervisor in a factory. She works very hard at her job, and is successful at it, but she is not content and always feels she ought to have done better. When other people do things wrong she takes the blame herself.

- Pine to help her know her real value, so that she can put aside unnecessary guilt.

We are all healers, and with love and sympathy in our natures we are also able to help anyone who really desires health.

THE ORIGINAL WRITINGS

Answers to revision exercise 1

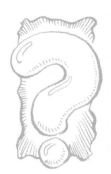

1. If you keep making the same mistakes you might need Chestnut Bud.

2. Rock Water people are very strict with themselves.

3. Someone who always laughs off problems instead of facing them needs Agrimony.

4. The worst kind of ultimate despair and unbearable anguish calls for Sweet Chestnut.

5. People who get depressed when things go a bit wrong need Gentian.

6. Rock Rose is the remedy for sheer terror.

7. When you know what you want to do but don't trust your own decision you need Cerato.

8. People in a Holly state suffer from very negative feelings towards others, like envy, hatred, suspicion and revengeful thoughts.

9. Beech people criticise others and find it difficult to be tolerant of other ways of life.

10. If you are living in the past you need Honeysuckle.

Revision exercise 2

Sometimes people get confused between particular pairs of remedies. Look at the following situations and decide which of the remedies given in brackets would be most appropriate in each case. As usual, the answers – and an explanation for the choice made – can be found on the following page.

1. All I've ever wanted was a husband, a home and a family. But I can't make up my mind whether I want to marry George or not. (CERATO or SCLERANTHUS or WILD OAT)

2. When I get into work and look at all the things there are to do I just feel exhausted. (HORNBEAM or OLIVE)

3. The past has such an influence over her – she makes no plans for the future, and hardly sees the present. (HONEYSUCKLE or WALNUT)

4. I always keep the house absolutely spotless – I'm terrified of dirt and some-times catch myself wiping the same table 20 or more times in a morning. (CRAB APPLE or ROCK WATER)

5. I want you to do things this way, not because I say so but because it's the right thing to do. (VERVAIN or VINE)

6. I can't stand having to work with her. She's just so slow! (BEECH or IMPATIENS)

7. There's no point talking to her – she's too busy dreaming of success to make it happen. (CLEMATIS or HONEYSUCKLE)

8. He's just given up all hope, but anyone can see that there might still be a way out of his troubles if only he'd make an effort. (GENTIAN or GORSE or MUSTARD or SWEET CHESTNUT)

9. He's a really brave man – he just laughs when you commiserate with him on his loss, and turns the whole thing into a huge joke. (AGRIMONY or OAK)

10. Ever since her children left home she's been gossiping to anyone who'll listen about her woes. She's becoming quite unpopular, I can tell you. (CHICORY or HEATHER)

Answers to revision exercise 2

1. The remedy for this lady is Scleranthus. It isn't Wild Oat because she knows what she wants. It isn't Cerato because Cerato people do make up their minds – it is only after they have done so that they begin to doubt their own judgement and look for confirmation.

2. It is the thought of starting work that causes the fatigue, and not the fact that work has been done. The correct remedy then is Hornbeam.

3. Although the talk of an outside influence might suggest Walnut, this person is living in the past and has no interest in present or future, which is a clear sign for Honeysuckle.

4. If Rock Water people keep the house spotless it is because they live by high standards – which is not the case here. This person's fear of contamination and obsessive behaviour both indicate Crab Apple.

5. Vine people would want things done their way regardless of right and wrong. The appeal to impersonal justice indicates Vervain.

6. Irritability like this would be Beech if it were the other person's mannerisms or way of life that were the trigger. In this case it is specifically slowness that is complained of, and like many Impatiens people this person seems to prefer working alone so that he can work at his own pace.

– CASE HISTORY –

Neil is an easy-going sort of person with no real ambitions, and happy in a humdrum job. When he is unexpectedly made redundant he seems to accept that as well, but as weeks stretch into months without a new job coming along he begins to feel that life might be passing him by.

- Wild Rose to help him to take more control over and feel more interested in his life.

7. Honeysuckle and Clematis people can both be inattentive — the fact that this lady's daydreams are of possible future happiness indicates Clematis.

8. If he had simply become discouraged, it would be Gentian; if there were no reason for being depressed, it would be Mustard; and if there really was no way out of present trouble, despite every effort having been made, then it would be Sweet Chestnut. As it is, this is a clear case for Gorse.

9. The Oak person can face up to pain and torment and keep going just the same — but here the attempt to minimise torment in sometimes inappropriate ways would suggest Agrimony instead.

10. Neither Chicory nor Heather people like being alone, but Chicory people are stronger and tend to focus on the ones they love. This lady is probably a Heather since she is trying to gain *any* audience and seems quite forgetful of her own self-respect along the way.

The Bach Centre today

Over the years the house at Mount Vernon and the people who worked there became known all over the world as the Dr Edward Bach Centre, or the Bach Centre for short. The trustees of the Centre were Dr Bach's co-workers Nora and Victor, who passed on their responsibilities to John Ramsell and Nickie Murray. Nickie decided to retire in the mid-eighties, and John asked his daughter Judy Howard to join the team, which she did.

John and Judy are still the trustees at the Bach Centre. Along with a team of half a dozen others they continue to make all the mother tinctures for the Bach Flower Remedies, and to give free help and advice to anyone who cares to ask for it. Visitors arrive in the village of Sotwell from all over the world, just to see Dr Bach's home and the furniture he made and of course his garden.

The Bach Centre has remained

> **DR BACH'S WISHES**
>
> 'This work of healing has been done, and published and given freely so that people like yourselves can help yourselves' — Edward Bach in a lecture in Wallingford, 24th September 1936.
>
> 'Our work is steadfastly to adhere to the simplicity and purity of this method of healing' — Edward Bach in a letter to Victor Bullen, 26th October 1936.
>
> (Both reprinted in The Orginal Writings of Edward Bach).

a completely independent organisation. It is not owned by any commercial company and has as its unique aim the continuation, protection and furtherance of Dr Bach's wishes, both as regards his work and the effect he wanted it to have in the world. From Sotwell the message of true healing goes all over the world: the power to heal really does lie in the hands of each and every one of us.

Final quiz

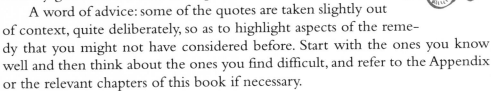

You will find that the best description of Dr Bach's 38 remedies is in his own book *The Twelve Healers*. On this and the next three pages there are 38 short quotations from each of his 38 remedy descriptions and the names of all 38 remedies. But they are muddled up: it's up to you to decide which remedy goes with which description.

A word of advice: some of the quotes are taken slightly out of context, quite deliberately, so as to highlight aspects of the remedy that you might not have considered before. Start with the ones you know well and then think about the ones you find difficult, and refer to the Appendix or the relevant chapters of this book if necessary.

ROCK ROSE

MIMULUS

CHERRY PLUM

ASPEN

RED CHESTNUT

CERATO

SCLERANTHUS

GENTIAN

GORSE

HORNBEAM

WILD OAT

CLEMATIS

HONEYSUCKLE

WILD ROSE

OLIVE

WHITE CHESTNUT

MUSTARD

CHESTNUT BUD

WATER VIOLET

IMPATIENS

HEATHER

AGRIMONY

CENTAURY

WALNUT

HOLLY

LARCH

PINE

ELM

SWEET CHESTNUT

STAR OF BETHLEHEM

WILLOW

OAK

CRAB APPLE

CHICORY

VERVAIN

VINE

BEECH

ROCK WATER

Fears, for which there can be given no explanation, no reason.

Gives constancy and protection from outside influences.

Unhappy if they have to be alone.

Suffer much from being unable to decide between two things.

They have a great wish to convert all around them.

The remedy of emergency.

Those who for a time refuse to be consoled.

Over-anxious to serve others.

Although their ambitions are strong, they have no calling.

Fear of worldly things.

For the different forms of vexation.

They desire that those for whom they care should be near them.

They do not expect further happiness such as they have had.

Wish all things to be done without hesitation or delay.

Any small delay or hindrance to progress causes doubt.

There is nothing but destruction and annihilation left to face.

They constantly seek advice from others, and are often misguided.

They are hard masters to themselves.

They judge life much by the success which it brings.

For those of whom they are fond they may suffer much.

They feel that the task they have undertaken is too difficult.

Even in illness they will direct their attendants.

Quiet people ... living more in the future than in the present.

They are aloof, leave people alone and go their own way.

They will fight on.

They hide their cares behind their humour.

Fear ... of reason giving way.

They feel they have no more strength to make any effort.

They have surrendered to the struggle of life without complaint.

As though a cold dark cloud overshadowed them and hid the light and joy of life.

Those who feel the need to see more good and beauty in all that surrounds them.

Thoughts which worry and will remain, or if for a time thrown out, will return.

Suffer much from the faults they attach to themselves.

Feel as if they had something not quite clean about themselves.

Do not consider themselves as good or capable as those around them.

Those who do not take full advantage of observation and experience.

The affairs of every day seem too much for them to accomplish.

They have given up belief that more can be done for them.

— CASE HISTORY —

Yasmine has reached the end of her tether. She has been alone all weekend in her empty flat, and has quite calmly and rationally considered, and rejected, the idea of suicide. If it weren't for the fact that it would devastate her parents, she would do it, but even that way out is denied her and everything is black and without the least shred of hope.

- Sweet Chestnut for her anguish and sense of utter despair.

Answer to final quiz

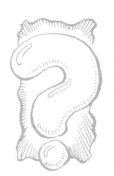

ROCK ROSE – the remedy of emergency

MIMULUS – fear of worldly things

CHERRY PLUM – fear … of reason giving way

ASPEN – fears, for which there can be given no explanation, no reason

RED CHESTNUT – for those of whom they are fond they may suffer much

CERATO – they constantly seek advice from others, and are often misguided

SCLERANTHUS – suffer much from being unable to decide between two things

GENTIAN – any small delay or hindrance to progress causes doubt

GORSE – they have given up belief that more can be done for them

HORNBEAM – the affairs of every day seem too much for them to accomplish

WILD OAT – although their ambitions are strong, they have no calling

CLEMATIS – quiet people … living more in the future than in the present

HONEYSUCKLE – they do not expect further happiness such as they have had

WILD ROSE – they have surrendered to the struggle of life without complaint

OLIVE – they feel they have no more strength to make any effort

WHITE CHESTNUT – thoughts which worry and will remain, or if for a time thrown out, will return

MUSTARD – as though a cold dark cloud overshadowed them and hid the light and joy of life

CHESTNUT BUD – those who do not take full advantage of observation and experience

WATER VIOLET – they are aloof, leave people alone and go their own way

IMPATIENS – wish all things to be done without hesitation or delay

HEATHER – unhappy if they have to be alone

AGRIMONY – they hide their cares behind their humour

CENTAURY – over-anxious to serve others

WALNUT – gives constancy and protection from outside influences

HOLLY – for the different forms of vexation

LARCH – do not consider themselves as good or capable as those around them

PINE – suffer much from the faults they attach to themselves

ELM – they feel that the task they have undertaken is too difficult

SWEET CHESTNUT – there is nothing but destruction and annihilation left to face

STAR OF BETHLEHEM – those who for a time refuse to be consoled

WILLOW – they judge life much by the success which it brings

OAK – they will fight on

CRAB APPLE – feel as if they had something not quite clean about themselves

CHICORY – they desire that those for whom they care should be near them

VERVAIN – they have a great wish to convert all around them

VINE – even in illness they will direct their attendants

BEECH – those who feel the need to see more good and beauty in all that surrounds them

ROCK WATER – they are hard masters to themselves

Now we've done ...

Remember the dwarves? Doc gave remedies to four of them, namely:

- Agrimony for Happy.

- Clematis for Sleepy.

- Mimulus for Bashful.

- Willow for Grumpy.

And he couldn't decide what to give Sneezy because he only had a physical symptom to go on ...

WHERE TO GO FROM HERE

Learning more about the Bach Flower Remedies

Although the Bach Flower Remedies are simple, human nature isn't. Even if you are already confident about your knowledge of the remedies, then, there is a lot more to learn. Fortunately there are a number of ways you can extend your knowledge.

BOOKS, VIDEOS AND CASSETTES

If you've come this far with this book you have already demonstrated that the self-study route is one you are good at. You can go on from here in the same way by using the books, videos or cassettes available through Bach Flower Remedy stockists or direct from the Bach Centre itself.

Books:
(All books are published by The C.W. Daniel Co. They can be ordered from local book shops or direct from the Bach Centre.)

- *The Twelve Healers and Other Remedies* by Dr Edward Bach – the one book that everyone should have, this gives the remedy indications in Dr Bach's own words and is the final authority.

- *Bach Flower Remedies Step by Step* by Judy Howard – a handy pocket-sized guide to the remedies and their use, complete with tips for selecting the right remedies at the right time.

- *Handbook of the Bach Flower Remedies* by Phillip Chancellor – detailed indications and case histories for each of the remedies, adapted by the author from the original writings of Nora Weeks.

- *Bach Flower Remedies for Women* by Judy Howard – a chronological survey of a woman's life with suggestions for using the remedies at each stage.

- *Bach Flower Remedies for Men* by Stefan Ball – the companion volume to *Women*, dealing with everything from babyhood and school exams to sex, work and retirement.

- *Growing Up with Bach Flower Remedies* by Judy Howard – to complete the Bach family, a guide to selecting remedies for children, from babyhood to adolescence.

- *Questions and Answers* by John Ramsell – a treasure trove of information on all aspects of Dr Bach's work, from the pronunciation of his name to the subtle differences between remedy pairs.

- *Heal Thyself* by Dr Edward Bach – the philosophy of healing that underpins practical work with the remedies, by Dr Bach himself.

- *The Original Writings of Edward Bach* edited by John Ramsell and Judy Howard – a selection of Dr Bach's writings from his early days in London right up to his last letters to his successors Nora and Victor.

- *The Medical Discoveries of Edward Bach, Physician* by Nora Weeks – a history of Dr Bach's professional life and of the remedies he discovered.

Cassettes

- *Getting to Know the Bach Flower Remedies* is a useful *aide-mémoire* published by the Bach Centre: side one contains descriptions of all 38 remedies, while side two provides exercises for practice – and gives you the answers as well!

Videos

- *Bach Flower Remedies: A Further Understanding* is a video produced by the Bach Centre which features interviews with the trustees who explain in a simple and straightfoward way how the remedies should be used.

- *The Light That Never Goes Out* is another Bach centre video, this time telling the story of Dr Bach's life and works and how both found a permanent home at Mount Vernon.

Healing yourself, your friends and your family

As well as consolidating your knowledge by reading you can go on with your practical work as well – this is one area of life where practice really does make perfect. The easiest way to get to know the remedies intimately is to use them yourself – and not, of course, only when you are ill. Dr Bach wanted the remedies to be part of everyday life, so if you feel worried take White Chestnut, and mix a couple of drops of Larch when you don't feel confident about things. This simple, everyday use of the remedies will not only help you to stay well-balanced and healthy, but it will teach you about yourself and about the way the remedies work in a more profound way than any book or video ever can.

Feel free to help your friends and relations as well. Of course, not everyone will want to try them and you might have to put up with the occasional sceptic. But you might be pleasantly surprised at how open most people are – and you may also discover that more people already use the remedies than you would have thought possible. Rescue Remedy in particular is a good way of introducing people to the benefits of the remedies, because in a crisis people are more prepared to accept help without criticising it beforehand. Once they have experienced for themselves how useful Rescue Remedy is they will be more inclined to listen when you tell them about the subtler effects of the whole range.

As for you, the effort of selecting for other people will also help teach you more about human nature, and with practice you will become adept at spotting people's type remedies and tracing their changing moods. The same thing can be done when watching films and television programmes, of course – and you might want to revisit some of the projects and exercises in this book from time to time, to refresh the knowledge you have already gained.

Courses in the UK and elsewhere

The best thing about attending a good course in the Bach Flower Remedies is that you will get to meet like-minded people. To this end, even a simple introductory course can be a useful experience, as well as giving you the opportunity to ask any questions that you haven't found an answer to in books. Remember that this book has (I hope) given you the building blocks you need to discover the remedies – attending a course and meeting other people on the same path is a good way to start building for real.

In the UK, there are courses in the Bach Flower Remedies starting up all the time. Some are run by local authorities and further education colleges, some by private individuals or private schools and health centres. Some of the courses being offered are very good, some are definitely to be avoided. Fortunately many of the good ones are run by practitioners trained at the Bach Centre, or otherwise with the co-operation of the Bach Centre, so if you are not sure whether a particular course is worth attending the best thing to do is to phone the Centre staff who will be pleased to tell you what they know.

There is in addition an official training programme, which is taught on two levels – introductory and advanced workshop. This is organised jointly by the Dr Edward Bach Foundation and A. Nelson & Co. Ltd, and full details are available on request from the Bach Centre.

Outside the UK, the Dr Edward Bach Foundation and A. Nelson & Co. Ltd are working together to bring the same official training programme to every country in the world. At the time of writing (February 1997) course have been run or are about to be run in the USA, Spain, Holland, Brazil and Canada. Again, the Bach Centre is your first contact point for more information on this aspect of the work. Other local courses outside the official programme may also be available – again, the Bach Centre may be able to recommend a contact point if you are having trouble finding a course where you live.

One word of warning might be added about correspondence courses. Many of these provide little in the way of tutor support, while the course workbooks contain a great deal less information than this one does – but you can easily pay more than £150 before you find this out. Some correspondence courses even offer 'diplomas' – but what they don't tell you is that these certificates are not recognised by any of the authoritative awarding bodies or by the Bach Centre or the Dr Edward Bach Foundation. They may look nice on the wall, but to genuine therapists these pieces of paper are taken more as a warning than a recommendation. If you are concerned to gain real recognition of your ability to use Dr Bach's system you might want to consider following a recognised practitioner training course which will lead to registration with the Dr Edward Bach Foundation.

Becoming a practitioner

You won't make your fortune by setting up as a professional practitioner in the Bach Flower Remedies. If you are doing your job properly you are teaching your clients how to use the remedies for themselves: the more successful you are, then, the less often your clients will need to come and see you. Nevertheless many people find real pleasure in being able to help strangers in this way, and of course the Bach Flower Remedies are a perfect accompaniment to other therapeutic practices such as aromatherapy, massage, reflexology and homoeopathy.

The Dr Edward Bach Foundation and its representatives administer a world-wide register of practitioners who have been trained to use Dr Bach's system. All of the people on its list have attended an approved course run either at the Bach Centre or at one of the approved training establishments scattered throughout the world. In addition they have all signed a Code of Practice which commits them to a caring and professional approach to their clients and to the protection of the purity, simplicity and completeness of Dr Bach's work.

The official practicioner course consists of four days in a classroom, followed by several months of coursework and by the prparation of detailed case studies showing the treatment over time of real-life clients. All stages of the course are thoroughly assessed. People who have demonstrated a thorough knowledge of the remedies and the ability to use them to help real people are then given the opportunity to apply for a place on the register.

If you want to go on a practitioner course write to the Dr Edward Bach Centre who will send you details of the courses nearest to you. The address is in the Appendix.

Appendix

Checklist of the 38 remedies

AGRIMONY	For mental torment hidden behind a smiling face
ASPEN	For fear or anxiety with no known cause
BEECH	For intolerance of other people and their behaviour and views
CENTAURY	For willing servants who find it hard to say 'no'
CERATO	For those who distrust their own judgement
CHERRY PLUM	For loss of control and the fear of doing harm to oneself or to others
CHESTNUT BUD	For repeated errors and the inability to learn from experience
CHICORY	For selfish, possessive, overbearing love
CLEMATIS	For day-dreaming, and living in an idealised future rather than the everyday present
CRAB APPLE	For dislike of one's own appearance or behaviour; for the cleansing of body and mind
ELM	For the crisis of confidence caused by taking on too much responsibility
GENTIAN	For discouragement and despondency caused by a setback
GORSE	For unjustified hopelessness, despair and defeatism
HEATHER	For self-obsessed people who talk constantly of their own affairs and need an audience
HOLLY	For negative feelings towards others such as hatred, jealousy, suspicion and spite
HONEYSUCKLE	For living in the past
HORNBEAM	For tiredness at the thought of the tasks that lie ahead

IMPATIENS	For impatience
LARCH	For lack of confidence that prevents attempts at success
MIMULUS	For everyday fear and anxiety caused by known things; also for shyness and timidity
MUSTARD	For gloom and depression with no known cause
OAK	For strong people who struggle on past the limits of their strength
OLIVE	For tiredness after great effort
PINE	For guilt and the tendency to blame oneself for everything that goes wrong
RED CHESTNUT	For fear that something awful will happen to loved ones
ROCK ROSE	For terror and extreme fear
ROCK WATER	For extreme self-control and mental rigidity
SCLERANTHUS	For the inability to choose between alternatives
STAR OF BETHLEHEM	For shock, and grief caused by loss
SWEET CHESTNUT	For ultimate despair, when everything is unutterly bleak and there is no way out
VERVAIN	For over-enthusiasm in a cause
VINE	For dominant people who rule others with a rod of iron
WALNUT	For protection against change and outside influences
WATER VIOLET	For private people who can appear proud or aloof
WHITE CHESTNUT	For constant, repetitive, worrying thoughts

WILD OAT	For uncertainty about what to do with one's life
WILD ROSE	For apathy and too easy acceptance of everything that happens
WILLOW	For self-pity, resentment and the blaming of others
RESCUE REMEDY	A mix of remedies used to deal with the immediate effects of crises, emergencies, attacks of nerves etc.
RESCUE CREAM	A mix of crisis remedies in a cream for external application where there is physical trauma

Useful addresses

Information on the remedies and their use, and referral to registered practitioners and training opportunities in the UK and throughout the world:

The Dr Edward Bach Centre
Mount Vernon
Bakers Lane
Sotwell
Oxon
OX10 0PZ
England
Tel: 01491 834678
Fax: 01491 825022
Email: centre@bachcentre.com
Website: www.bachcentre.com

Sales of Bach Flower Remedies and information on local availability throughout the world (except USA):

Bach Flower Remedies Customer Services
A Nelson & Co
Broadheath House
83 Parkside
London
SW19 5LP
England
Tel: 0181 780 4200

All sales and educational information for the USA:

Nelson Bach USA Ltd
100 Research Drive
Wilmington
MA 01887
USA
Tel   (Sales)   1 508 988 3833
Tel   (Education) 1 800 334 0843

Index

Page numbers in bold indicate the main reference for individual remedies

accidents and Bach
    remedies 32, 88
addresses 185
Agrimony 35, **108**
alternative medicine 86-7
anger 91, 109
animals: treatment 156-8
anxiety 23, 64
Aspen 23, **24-5**
  preparation 78

Bach, Dr Edward 27-9,
    52-3, 114-15, 141
  works
    Heal Thyself 86, 122, 175
    Original Writings 86,
      148, 163, 175
    Twelve Healers 11, 72,
      88, 90, 154, 174
Bach Centre 163-4
  resources 174-5
  training 176-7
Ball, Stefan 174
Beech 66, 68, **69**, 77, 112
body language 133-4
booklist 174-5
Bullen, Victor 141-2, 163

cassettes on Bach remedies
    175
categories of remedies *see*
    type remedies
Centaury **107-8**
Cerato **48-9**, 124
Chancellor, Phillip 174
character types *see* type
    remedies
checklist of remedies 182-4
Cherry Plum **25**, 44, 50, 154
Chestnut Bud 150, **151**

Chicory 68, **69-71**, 157
Clematis 44, 53, 107, 138,
    149
combination remedies 31,
    34, 148 *see also* Rescue
    Remedy
complementary medicine
    86
  Bach remedies as 26, 32,
    87, 88
confidence, lack of 123,
    124
consultations, conducting
    128-32, 137-9, 144
  and explaining remedy
    selection 139-41
courses in Bach remedies
    176-7
Crab Apple 45, **124-5**, 129
  for animals/plants 157
crises *see* Rescue Remedy

despondency/despair:
    remedies 123-7
  exercise 127-8
  and uncertainty remedies
    49, 71
diary of moods 36-8
discovery of remedies 52-3
disease: imbalance as cause
    33
Dr Edward Bach Centre
    see Bach Centre
doctors *see* orthodox
    medicine
dosage 29, 33-4
  for animals/plants 156-7
  of Rescue Remedy 44
dropper bottles *see*
    treatment bottles

Elm **123-4**, 130, 133
  preparation 78
emergencies *see* Rescue
    Remedy
emotions *see also* moods
  and health 33, 86, 89-90,
    96
  hidden 74, 136
  identifying 112-14, 176
exercises 54-7, 93-6, 97-8
    see also under specific
    type remedies, *e.g.* fear,
    remedies for
  revision 159-62
exhaustion 48-9, 151

fear, remedies for 22-5
  exercises 26-7, 30-2
feelings *see* emotions;
    moods

Gentian **49**, 71
Gorse **49**, 73, 79, 157
guilt 126

hatred 108-9
health and emotions *see*
    under emotions
Heather **91-2**
holistic approach 33, 86-7,
    96-7
Holly 51, **108-9**, 112
homeopathy: and Bach 29,
    71-2
Honeysuckle, 73, 136, 140,
    149
hopelessness 49, 108
Hornbeam **48-9**, 129, 150,
    151
Howard, Judy 163, 174

hygiene: and treatment
bottles 34

Impatiens 44, 53, 64, **92**,
112, 128
indecision 46-7
injuries and Bach remedies
32, 88
insufficient interest in
present circumstances:
remedies 149-52
exercises 152-4, 155-6

knowing yourself *see* self-
discovery

Larch 116, **123**
length of treatment 135
listening skills 128-32, 144
see also body language;
consultations
loneliness, remedies for
91-3

metaphors: and Bach
remedies 90
Mimulus **22-3**, 24, 25, 53,
64, 74, 78
examples of use 35, 110,
112, 157
mood remedies
selecting: exercises 21-2,
90-1
and type remedies 64-5
moods, identifying 112,
176
projects/exercises 20,
36-8, 113-14
Mount Vernon 27, 53,
141-2
Bach Centre at 163-4
and remedy preparation 78

Murray, Nickie 163
Mustard **152**, 158

nosodes, Bach 71-2

Oak 64, **124**
Olive 14, 49, 76, 135, **151**
orthodox medicine 33, 86,
96, 122
and Bach remedies 32,
87, 88
over-care for welfare of
others: remedies 66-71
exercise 72-4
over-enthusiasm 67-8
over-sensitivity to
influences and ideas:
remedies 106-9

'patients': implications 122
personality types *see* type
remedies
physical problems: and
Bach remedies 32, 86,
88-9
exercise 87-8
Pine **125-6**, 136, 159
plants: treatment 156-7
possessiveness 70-1
preparation of remedies
78-9
'prescribing': implications
122
professional practice 138
training for 176-7

quizzes
final 164-9
quick 39-40, 59-60, 81-2,
99-101, 116-18, 143-4

Ramsell, John 163, 174

Red Chestnut **23-4**, 25,
110
registration 177
Rescue Cream **45**, 125
Rescue Remedy 14, 31,
44-5
for animals/plants 156-7
examples of use 25, 56,
107
exercises 45-6, 57-8
quick results of 135,
175-6
resources 174-5
Rock Rose **25**, 44
Rock Water **69**, 69, 111

Scleranthus **46**, 48, 92
selection of remedies,
explaining 139-41
self-absorption 91-2
self-control, fear of losing
25
self-discovery 74, 104
projects 20, 105, 115-16
self-help, remedies as
122-3, 163
shyness 23, 64
simplicity of remedies 90,
148, 154, 163
Sotwell 141, 163
Star of Bethlehem 44, 56,
107, **127**, 157
sterilisation of bottles 34,
35-6
stock bottles 14, 29, 78
stress: exercise 110-12
suicide 25, 26
Sweet Chestnut **126-7**, 167

taking remedies: methods
29, 33-4, 44-5
tension, mental/physical 86

timidity 23, 64
tiredness 48-9, 151
training, professional 176-7
treatment bottles 29, 33-6,
    44
  and length of treatment
    135
type remedies 64-6
  identifying 74, 176
    exercises/projects 75-7,
    79-80, 90-1, 105, 115-
    16
  origin of 71-2

uncertainty, remedies for
    46-9
  exercise 50-2

Vervain **66-8**, 69, 86, 88,
    112, 151
videos on Bach remedies
    175
Vine **69**, 74, 79, 112

Wallingford: 1936 lecture
    148, 163
Walnut **106-7**, 108, 110, 140
  for animals/plants 157
Water Violet 72, **93**, 112,
    157
Weeks, Nora 53, 141-2,
    163, 175
welfare of others, over-care
    for: remedies 66-71
  exercise 72-4

White Chestnut 14, 110,
    150, 151
Wild Oat **47**, 52
Wild Rose **150-1**, 162
Willow 109, 114, **126**, 136,
    157
  preparation 78
worry 150